Pediatric Emergency Skills

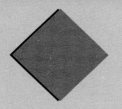

Pediatric Emergency Skills

Jill P. French, RN, MSN, CCRN
Project Director/Educational Consultant,
Pediatric Emergency Nurse Education Project;
Clinical Instructor,
Continuing Education Department,
School of Nursing,
University of North Carolina at Chapel Hill,
Chapel Hill, North Carolina

with 150 illustrations

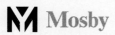 Mosby

St. Louis Baltimore Boston Carlsbad Chicago Naples New York
Philadelphia Portland London Madrid Mexico City Singapore

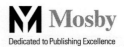

Mosby

Dedicated to Publishing Excellence

A Times Mirror Company

Editor-in-chief: Nancy Coon
Editor: Robin Carter
Assistant Editor: Kerri Rabbitt
Project Manager: Dana Peick
Production Editor: Cindy Deichmann
Designer: Jeanne Wolfgeher
Electronic Production Coordinator: Pamela Merritt
Manufacturing Manager: Betty Richmond
Illustration concepts by: Brian Kennedy
Illustrations by: Ted Bolte
Cover Designer: Amy Buxton

Copyright © 1995 by Mosby–Year Book, Inc.

A NOTE TO THE READER
The authors and publisher have made every attempt to check dosages and nursing content for accuracy. Because the science of pharmacology is continually advancing, our knowledge base continues to expand. Therefore, we recommend that the reader always check product information for changes in dosage or administration before administering any medication. This is particularly important with new or rarely used drugs.

This book was developed as a special project of the School of Nursing Continuing Education Program at the University of North Carolina at Chapel Hill with assistance from the Kate B. Reynolds Health Care Trust.

Printed in the United States of America

Composition by Mosby Electronic Production, St. Louis
Printing/binding by Western Publishing

Mosby–Year Book, Inc.
11830 Westline Industrial Drive
St. Louis, Missouri 63146

International Standard Book Number 0-8151-3358-8

95 96 97 98 99 / 9 8 7 6 5 4 3 2 1

Contributors

Tina Adams, RN
Pediatric Transport Nurse,
University of North Carolina Children's Hospital,
Chapel Hill, North Carolina
> Temperature Assessment
> Using Radiant Warmers
> Using an Isolette

Kirsten Johnson Moore, RN, MSN
Staff Nurse,
Medical Intensive Care Unit,
Children's Hospital,
Boston, Massachusetts
> Intraosseous Needle Insertion
> Securing Intraosseous Needle
> Administration of Oxygen
> Placing an Indwelling Urinary Catheter
> Securing an Indwelling Urinary Catheter

Wren Wallace, RN, BSN, CCRN
Nurse Education Clinician,
Pediatric Intensive Care Unit,
University of North Carolina Children's Hospital,
Chapel Hill, North Carolina
> Bag-Valve-Mask Ventilation
> Ventilation via an Endotracheal or Tracheostomy Tube
> Suctioning
> Securing an Endotracheal Tube
> Medication Delivery via an Endotracheal Tube

Illustration Concepts and Instructional Design

Brian G. Kennedy, BFA, MFA
Artist and Proprietor of BK Design Co.,
Carrboro, North Carolina

Nancy E. Kiplinger, MEd
Design and Educational Support Center,
School of Nursing,
University of North Carolina at Chapel Hill,
Chapel Hill, North Carolina

Acknowledgments

The author and contributors are very appreciative for the review and comments given by the following individuals during the development of the manual.

Tina Adams, RN
Pediatric Transport Nurse,
University of North Carolina Children's Hospital,
Chapel Hill, North Carolina

Lela Brink, MD
Acting Chief,
Pediatric Critical Care Division;
Director,
Pediatric Intensive Care Unit,
University of North Carolina Children's Hospital,
Chapel Hill, North Carolina

Warren Crow, RN, BSN
Nurse Manager,
Emergency Department,
Moses H. Cone Memorial Hospital,
Greensboro, North Carolina

Karen Frush, MD
Assistant Clinical Professor,
Department of Pediatrics;
Director,
Pediatric Emergency Medicine,
Duke University Medical Center,
Durham, North Carolina

Susan Hohenhaus, RN, CEN
Nurse Education Clinician,
Emergency Department,
University of North Carolina Hospitals,
Chapel Hill, North Carolina

Arlene Jacobs, RN, BSN
Director,
The Hemby Pediatric Trauma Institute,
Carolinas Medical Center,
Charlotte, North Carolina

Kirsten Johnson Moore, RN, MSN
Staff Nurse,
Medical Intensive Care Unit,
Children's Hospital,
Boston, Massachusetts

Crela Landreth, RN
President,
North Carolina Emergency Nurses' Association,
Trauma Coordinator,
Memorial Mission Hospital,
Asheville, North Carolina

Sarah S. Norwood, RN, MSN
Educational Consultant,
North Carolina Emergency Medical Services for Children Project,
University of North Carolina Hospitals,
Chapel Hill, North Carolina

Lew Romer, MD
Assistant Professor,
Department of Pediatrics;
Director,
Pediatric Critical Care Fellowship Program,
University of North Carolina Children's Hospital,
Chapel Hill, North Carolina

Developmental guidelines also reviewed by:

Cathee J. Huber, RN, MN, PhD Candidate
Developmental Nursing Specialist and Director of Training,
The Clinical Center for the Study of Development and Learning,
University of North Carolina at Chapel Hill,
Chapel Hill, North Carolina

A special thanks to **Martha Petersen**, Continuing Education Department at the University of North Carolina at Chapel Hill, for her contributions in word processing and organizing.

Consultants

The following consultants served as reviewers:

Deborah A. Kotrada, RN, CEN
Dartmouth-Hitchcock Medical Center
Hanover, NH

Renee Semonin Holleran, RN, PhD, CEN, CCRN, CFRN
Chief Flight Nurse
University Air Care
University of Cincinnati
Cincinnati, OH

Pamela S. Kidd, RN, PhD, CEN
Assistant Professor
College of Nursing
University of Kentucky
Lexington, KY

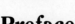

Preface

The purpose of this manual is to provide well-illustrated and thorough guidelines for the performance of nursing procedures for infants and children. This manual is written for emergency department nurses, clinic nurses, transport nurses, pediatric nurses, students of nursing, and nurses who may infrequently care for pediatric patients.

The manual consists of guidelines for specific pediatric techniques and accompanying case studies that exemplify application of the procedures. The guidelines for each technique, with a few exceptions, are all written in the following format: (1) Purpose; (2) Supplies; and (3) Procedure, with illustrations to clarify specific steps of the procedure. The reader will find developmental guidelines in the last section; these are intended to be incorporated into each procedural guideline.

Before performing any procedure, a nurse should be familiar with his or her institutional policy and procedure manual, as well as the Nurse Practice Act for that state. Although this manual offers guidelines based on relevant research, the policies and procedures of individual institutions must be followed. These guidelines may be helpful when revising older policies or may serve as standards where written policies are not available.

Case studies are designed to integrate didactic information and technical skills. Case study questions are intended to stimulate discussion and to encourage learners to demonstrate skills.

This manual provides a clinical reference tool and a framework for teaching pediatric skills. It is intended for clinical use and to accompany interactive teaching. The manual may be used for teaching in several ways: in workshop format, for educational inservices, or during individual precepting. The illustrated guidelines, in conjunction with hands-on practice and case study discussion, will prepare nurses to care for critically ill or injured children.

Jill French

Contents

Stabilization Procedures 135

Developmental Issues 177

Case Studies 197

Appendixes 241

Pediatric Emergency Skills

CHAPTER

1

Venous Access

Blood Sample Collection

➤ **PURPOSE**

    To identify blood sample collection sites and apply appropriate techniques for drawing venous, arterial, and capillary blood samples in pediatric patients.

➤ **SUPPLIES**

Nonsterile gloves
Warm, wet towel or commercial heat pack
Alcohol pads
Povidone-iodine solution
2″ x 2″ gauze pads
Sterile adhesive bandage strips

Specific for venipuncture and arterial puncture:
23 gauge butterfly needle or 25 gauge straight needle
Three 10 ml syringes
Blood collection tubes
Heparinized syringe* (for arterial puncture)
Ice-filled container (for arterial puncture)
Tourniquet or rubber band to use as tourniquet (for
    venipuncture)

Specific for capillary sample:
Microlancet
Blood collection tubes (capillary tubes)
Clay sealer

➤ **GENERAL PROCEDURES**

1. Assemble equipment. Keep needles out of the child's sight.

---

*If ready-to-use heparinized syringes are not available, prepare a 1 ml or 3 ml syringe by drawing heparin (any concentration) into the cylinder. Coat the inside of the cylinder and expel the solution.

2. Procure assistance to restrain the infant or child.

3. Explain to the child and family the need for blood sample collection.
   Be honest; tell the child that it will hurt and you will do it quickly. Tell the child it's all right to cry. Ask him or her to try to hold still.

   - *If the child is 2 to 7 years old, tell him or her right before you are ready to start.*

   - *If the child is older and time permits, tell him or her 5 to 10 minutes before beginning the procedure.*

4. Offer parents the option of staying for the procedure or waiting outside.
   Some parents may need permission to leave. If they stay, their role is to offer support, not to restrain the child.[1,2]

5. Wash hands.

➤ *PROCEDURE—Venipuncture*

Used to obtain blood samples for blood chemistry analysis, hematologic values, and serum drug concentrations.

Follow Steps 1 through 5 of the General Procedure, then:

6. Explain to the child that you are "just looking" now and that you will tell him or her before you do anything.[1]

7. Identify potential venipuncture sites. Consider the age of the child, the illness or injury the child has sustained, and the specific anatomical characteristics of the child. Potential sites are based on age, as shown in Table 1-1.

8. Use a tourniquet and palpate to select site. Table 1-2 lists the sites and gives suggestions for locating and using them.

Table 1-1	Venipuncture Sites	
Infant: < 1 year	**Toddler: 1 - 3 years**	**Child: > 3 years**
antecubital fossa	antecubital fossa	antecubital fossa
hand	hand	hand
foot	foot	
scalp		

Table 1-2	Locating Venipuncture Sites
Location	**Procedure/Explanation**
Antecubital fossa	• This is the most accessible site for obtaining venous blood in children of all ages.[3] • **Location:** Basilic and cephalic veins branch out to form an M; any of these veins may be used. • **To use:** Extend and supinate the child's forearm; veins will "bounce" when palpated.
Hand	• Hand veins are often quite visible but not well anchored and tend to roll. • **Location:** Basilic and cephalic veins branch across the dorsum of the hand; the cephalic vein ("intern's vein") travels along the lateral part of the hand and is often easily cannulated, but any of the hand's veins may be used. • **To use:** Pronate the hand and flex at the wrist.
Foot	• Foot veins may be used if the infant or toddler will not be ambulatory. • **Location:** The great saphenous vein lies one finger's breadth up and over from the medial malleolus; the lateral and medial marginal veins may also be used. • **To use:** Extend the foot at the ankle so that the toes point downward.
Scalp	• Scalp veins may be used if other sites are poor. (Using a scalp vein may be considered an infection risk if the infant is under the care of a neurologist or neurosurgeon. Consult with the service before using a scalp vein.) • **Location:** Any of the superficial veins of the scalp may be used; distinguish veins from arteries, as these lie close together on the scalp. • **To use:** Apply a rubber band as a tourniquet* around the forehead and occiput; before placing the rubber band on the scalp, wrap a piece of tape on it to allow for quick removal.

* Before applying tourniquet, shave the scalp around the selected vein; save the hair for the parents. (Let the parents know beforehand if a scalp vein is to be used and shaving is required.)

Anticubital Fossa

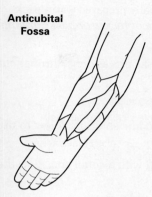

Hand

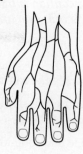

Foot

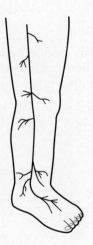

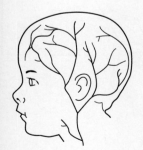

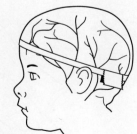

Scalp

9. If using the antecubital fossa, hand, or foot, warm the site with a warm, wet towel or a commercially prepared warm pack. *Use caution with the temperature of towels or packs; infants have thin skin and burn easily.*

10. Put on gloves. Maintain universal precautions throughout the procedure.

11. Reapply the tourniquet.

12. Cleanse the site with povidone-iodine solution. Allow to dry for 60 seconds.

13. Wipe povidone-iodine solution off with alcohol and allow the alcohol to dry.

14. Grasp the area distal to the site and pull slightly to stabilize the skin and veins.

15. Grasp the needle firmly.
    - If using a butterfly needle, pinch the butterfly wings together between thumb and forefinger.
    - If using a needle with syringe, hold it normally.

16. Insert the needle, bevel up, at a 30° to 45° angle 0.5 to 1.0 cm distal to the point where you expect the needle to enter the vein (Fig. 1-1).

Fig 1-1

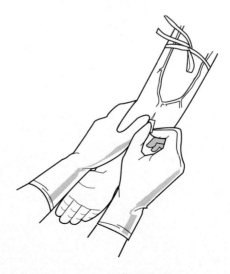

17. After piercing the skin, lower the catheter shaft to 10° to 15° and move the needle directly above the vein.

18. Enter the vein slowly, verifying entry by a flashback of blood.

19. Draw blood into the syringe. If using a butterfly needle, attach the syringe to the tubing and withdraw the plunger slowly. If using a straight needle, withdraw the syringe plunger slowly. *Withdrawing the plunger too quickly may cause the vein to collapse and blood flow to cease. If this occurs, release tension and slowly withdraw again.*

20. When the sample is complete, remove the tourniquet, cover the site with a gauze pad, and remove the needle. Apply pressure to the site.

21. Transfer the blood to the collection tubes.

22. Apply a bandage.

23. Give the child positive feedback.

➤ *PROCEDURE—Arterial Puncture*

Used to obtain blood samples for determining the partial pressure of gases.

Follow steps 1 through 5 of the General Procedure, then:

6. Explain to the child that you are "just looking" now and you will tell him or her before you do anything.[1]

7. Identify potential sites by palpation. The sites are described in Table 1-3.

Table 1-3 Locating Arterial Puncture Sites	
Location	**Procedure/Explanation**
Radial artery	• This is the preferred site for children of all ages because it contains collateral blood supply and is not close to the median nerve.[4] • **Location:** The ventral surface of the wrist at the skin creases. • **To use:** Flex the wrist over a gauze roll, palm side up.
Posterior tibial artery	• May be used if the radial artery is overused or indispensible. • **Location:** Posterior to the medial malleolus. • **To use:** Flex the foot; follow the path of the artery with your finger.
Dorsalis pedis artery	• May be used if the radial artery is overused or indispensible. • **Location:** The middle of the dorsum of the foot, between the ankle and the toes. • **To use:** Hold the foot in plantar flexion.

Radial artery

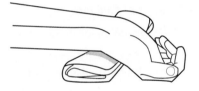

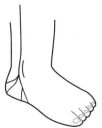

Posterior tibial artery

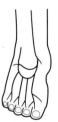

Dorsalis pedis artery

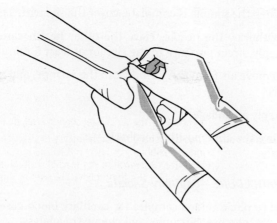

Fig 1-2

8. Put on gloves. Maintain universal precautions throughout the procedure.

9. Cleanse the area with povodine-iodine solution. Allow to dry for 60 seconds.

10. Wipe with alcohol and allow to dry.

11. Grasp the needle firmly.

   • If using a butterfly needle, pinch the butterfly wings together between thumb and first finger.
   • If using a needle with syringe, hold it normally.

12. Position the needle at a 45° angle 0.5 cm distal to the point of strongest pulsation and insert it swiftly (Fig. 1-2).

13. Once the needle has entered the skin, palpate the artery again and adjust the position of the needle.

14. If a flashback is not seen, slowly pull the needle back. Reposition and advance again.

15. Once a flashback is seen, steady the needle and have another health care provider pull the sample into the syringe.

16. When the sample is complete, cover the site with a gauze pad.

17. Withdraw the needle. Have the other health care provider apply direct pressure to the site for at least 5 minutes.

18. Remove air from the syringe, cap the syringe, and place it on ice.

19. Apply a bandage.

20. Give the child positive feedback.

➤ **PROCEDURE—*Capillary Sample***

Used to obtain blood samples for capillary blood gases, hematocrit, glucose, bilirubin, and chemistry analysis.

Follow steps 1 to 5 of the General Procedure, then:

6. Choose the finger or heel to stick.

   • If the child is ambulatory, the ventral lateral aspect of the fingertip is the best location (Fig. 1-3).
   • If the child is not ambulatory, use the heel (Fig. 1-4).
   The medial aspect of the heel is highly vascular and is a good site. The lateral aspect may also be used. Avoid the bottom of the heel where many nerves travel.

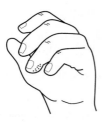

Fig 1-3

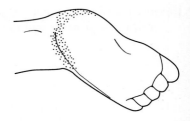

Fig 1-4

Fig 1-5

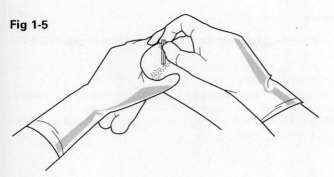

7. Warm the site with a warm, wet towel or a commercially-prepared warm pack.
   Be certain the temperature of the towel or pack is not too warm.

8. Put on gloves. Maintain universal precautions throughout the procedure.

9. Cleanse the site with alcohol and allow it to dry.

10. Using a swift motion and firm pressure, introduce the lancet at a 90° angle on the lateral aspect of the finger or sole of the foot[3] (Fig. 1-5).

11. Wipe the first drop of blood with a gauze pad.

12. Gently "milk" the extremity to allow blood to let.
    Be careful not to squeeze unnecessarily as the blood may hemolyze.

13. Hold the capillary tube at a 60° angle to the site and allow the blood sample to draw up the tube. Do not allow air to enter the sample.

14. When the tube is ¾ filled, place your finger over the distal end of the tube and place the other end of the tube in clay.
    If the sample is for capillary gas, seal and transport according to your institution's policy.

15. Apply a bandage.

16. Give the child positive feedback.

References

1 O'Brian R: Starting intravenous lines in children, *J Emerg Nurs* 17(4):225-230, 1991.
2 Campbell LS: Starting intravenous lines in children: tips for success, *J Emerg Nurs* 17(3):177-178, 1991.
3 Lynd M, Kesler RW: Blood collection procedures. In Lohr JA, ed.: *Pediatric outpatient procedures*, Philadelphia, 1991, JB Lippincott, pp. 258-274.
4 Suddaby EC, Sourbeer MO: Drawing pediatric arterial blood gases, *Crit Care Nurse* 10(7):28-31, 1990.

Peripheral Intravenous (IV) Cannulation

To identify venous cannulation sites rapidly and apply appropriate techniques for cannulation.

➤ **SUPPLIES**

Over-the-needle catheter
Nonsterile gloves
Warm, wet towel or commercial heat pack
Tourniquet or rubber band (for scalp veins)
Povidone-iodine solution
Alcohol pads
3 ml syringe filled with normal saline
T-connector
1/4" to 1/2" adhesive tape
Padded armboard
Razor (for scalp veins)
2"x 2" sterile gauze pads
Antiseptic ointment
Normal saline or heparin flush solution (10 U/ml)
IV infusion setup
IV infusion pump
IV fluids

➤ **PROCEDURE**

1. Assemble IV infusion setup and purge with the IV fluids ordered.

   • Ensure that there are no bubbles in the tubing.
   • Label the bag and tubing with date and time.
   • Place the end of tubing within easy reach.

2. Assemble cannulation supplies. Keep needles out of sight of the child.

   • Flush the T-connector with normal saline or heparin solution.
   • Ensure that there are no bubbles in the T-connector.
   • Place the T-connector within easy reach to immediately attach it to the catheter hub.

   The use of a T-connector decreases movement and tension on the catheter and allows for IV tubing change without disturbing the dressing or manipulating the catheter.[1,2]

3. Cut tape in 1 cm x 5 cm pieces for securing the IV catheter.

4. Procure assistance to restrain the infant or child.

5. Explain to the child and family the need for IV cannulation.

   • Be careful in your choice of words; for example, "IV" may be interpreted as "ivy" by the child.
   • Explain that you will put "a small tube in your arm" and that a needle is used in the beginning and then taken out and thrown away.
   • Be honest (tell the child that it will hurt and you will try to do it quickly).
   • If the child is 2 to 7 years old, tell him or her right before you are ready to start.
   • If the child is older and time permits, tell him or her 5 to 10 minutes before the cannulation attempt.

6. Ask the parent if the child has any known allergies (e.g., antiseptics, tape, medications).

7. Offer parents the option of staying for the procedure or waiting outside.
   Some parents may need permission to leave. If they do stay, their role is to offer support, not to restrain the child.[1,3]

8. Wash hands.

9. Explain to the child that you are "just looking" now and that you will tell him or her before you do anything.[1]

10. Identify potential cannulation sites. Consider the age of the child, the illness or injury the child has sustained, and the specific anatomical characteristics of the child. Potential sites are based on age, as shown in Table 1-4.

Table 1-4	Cannulation Sites	
Infant < 1 year	**Toddler 1 to 3 years**	**Child > 3 years**
hand	hand	hand
foot	foot	antecubital fossa
scalp	antecubital fossa	
antecubital fossa		

NOTE:

- Use distal sites first.
- Select a site that will least interfere with the child's developmental abilities.
- Avoid sites that limit mobility.
- Avoid the dominant hand.

11. Use a tourniquet and palpate to select site. Table 1-5 lists the sites and gives suggestions for locating and using them.

12. If using the hand or foot, prepare the site with commercially-prepared warm packs or a warm, wet towel.
Warming causes the vein to vasodilate and increases visibility.[1] Use caution with the temperature of the towels or packs; infants have thin skin and burn easily. Other techniques to increase visibility include placing the extremity in a dependent position and using a transillumination device.[4]

13. Select the appropriate size cannulation device (Box 1-1). Rotate the needle before insertion to release any seal it has on the catheter.

14. The site may be secured to an armboard before or after cannulation.

The armboard restricts mobility and should maintain the extremity in a natural anatomic position. The armboard can be explained to the child as a "pillow" for the hand or extremity.[1]

If cannulating veins in the antecubital area, tape the hand palm down; this facilitates stabilization of the site by forcing the child to use a weaker muscle as the flexor.[5]

Table 1-5	Locating Cannulation Sites
Location	**Procedure/Explanation**
Hand	• Veins are often quite visible but not well-anchored and tend to roll. • **Location:** Basilic and cephalic veins branch across the dorsum of the hand; the cephalic vein ("intern's vein") travels along the lateral part of the hand and is often easily cannulated, but any of the hand's veins may be used. • **To use:** Pronate the hand and flex at the wrist.
Foot	• Foot veins may be used if infant or toddler will not be ambulatory. • **Location:** The great saphenous vein lies one finger's breadth up and over from the medial malleolus; the lateral and medial marginal veins may also be used. • **To use:** Extend the foot at the ankle so that the toes point downward.
Scalp	• Scalp veins may be used if other sites are poor. (Using a scalp vein may be considered an infection risk if the infant is under care of a neurologist or neurosurgeon. Consult with the service before using a scalp vein.) • **Location:** Any of the superficial veins of the scalp may be used; distinguish veins from arteries, as both lie close together on the scalp. • **To use:** Apply a rubber band as a tourniquet* around the forehead and occiput; before placing the rubber band on the scalp, wrap a piece of tape on it to allow for quick removal.
Antecubital fossa	• Veins are difficult to immobilize after cannulation and often used for blood sample collection.[2] • **Location:** Basilic and cephalic veins branch out to form an M; any of these veins may be used. • **To use:** Extend and supinate the child's forearm; veins will "bounce" when palpated.

*Before applying tourniquet, shave the scalp around the selected vein; save the hair for the parents. (Let the parents know beforehand if a scalp vein is to be used and shaving is required.)

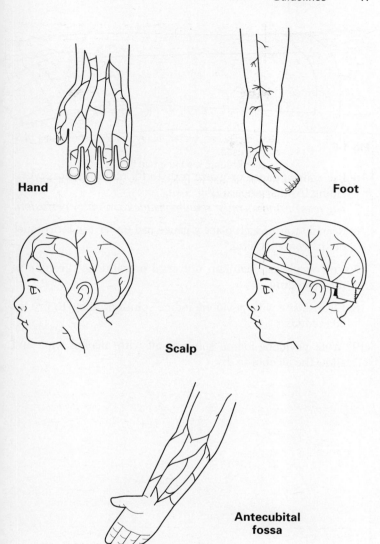

Hand

Foot

Scalp

**Antecubital
fossa**

Box 1-1 Over-the-Needle Catheters

24 or 22 gauge for infants < 1 year
22, 20, or 18 gauge for children 1 to 12 years
20, 18, or 16 gauge for children > 12 years

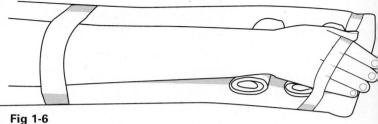

Fig 1-6

15. Use rolls of gauze or gauze pads to fill natural spaces when taping to an armboard (Fig. 1-6).
The toes or fingers must remain visible to monitor perfusion.

16. Reapply tourniquet; place a gauze pad under the tourniquet tie to avoid pinching.[6]

17. Put on gloves. Maintain universal precautions throughout the procedure.

18. Cleanse site with povidone-iodine solution. Allow to dry for 60 seconds.

19. Wipe povidone-iodine solution off with alcohol wipe and allow the alcohol to dry.

Fig 1-7

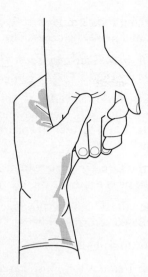

20. Grasp the area distal to the site and pull slightly to stabilize the skin and vein (Fig. 1-7).

21. Insert the needle, bevel up, at a 30° to 45° angle 0.5 to 1.0 cm distal to the site where you expect the needle to enter the vein (Fig. 1-8).

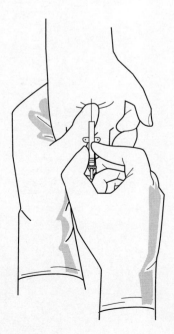

Fig 1-8

22. After piercing the skin, lower the catheter shaft to a 10° to 15° angle and move the needle directly above the vein.

    Entering from the side may cause the needle to perforate the vein as the width and depth of small veins are variable.[2]

23. Enter the vein slowly, verifying entry by flashback of blood. Once the flashback is seen, advance both the catheter and needle 1 to 3 mm further to ensure the catheter is inserted beyond the bevel.[5]

24. Advance the catheter while withdrawing the needle. Do not reinsert the needle into the catheter after it has been removed.

25. If possible, allow blood to flow back and fill the hub of the catheter. Blood return may be minimal in small veins.

26. Release the tourniquet.

27. Attach the T-connector. Flush carefully to determine patency. If the catheter was not advanced while withdrawing the needle, it may be advanced while flushing.

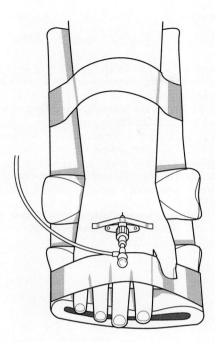

Fig 1-9

28. Apply one strip of tape (1 cm x 5 cm) across the catheter per-
    pendicularly to temporarily secure (Fig. 1-9). Tape catheter
    securely in place (see "Taping IV Catheters").

29. Connect immediately to a continuous infusion or flush with
    heparin solution (10 U/1 ml) to avoid clotting at the site from
    fibrin deposition.[1,7] Infuse room-temperature fluids.

30. Give the child positive feedback.

31. Document at the IV site the date, size of the catheter, and the
    initials of the person who started the IV.

32. Document in the notes the site of the catheter insertion, size
    of the catheter, the type and rate of IV infusion, and how the
    child tolerated the procedure.

References

[1] O'Brian R: Starting intravenous lines in children, *J Emerg Nurs* 17(4):225-230, 1991.

[2] Wilson D: Neonatal IVs: practical tips, *Neonatal Netw* 11(2):49-53, 1992.

[3] Campbell LS: Starting intravenous lines in children: tips for success, *J Emerg Nurs* 17(3):177-178, 1991.

[4] Blatz S, Paes BA: Intravenous infusion by superficial vein in the neonate, *J Intraven Nurs* 13(2):122-128, 1990.

[5] Norwood SS: IV access, fluids and medications. In Norwood SS, Zaritsky AL, eds.: *Guidelines to pediatric emergency care,* 1992, Emergency Medical Services for Children Project.

[6] Martin S: Procedures involving the cardiovascular system. In Bernardo L, Bove M, eds.: *Pediatric emergency nursing procedures,* Boston, 1993, Jones & Bartlett, pp. 83-123.

[7] Morrow JC: Simplifying nursing management of pediatric airways and intravenous infusions, *J Emerg Nurs* 14(2):103-106, 1988.

Taping Intravenous (IV) Catheters

➤ **PURPOSE**

To secure an IV catheter appropriately to prevent dislodgement and enhance ongoing observation of the site.

➤ **SUPPLIES**

Nonsterile gloves
$\frac{1}{4}$" to $\frac{1}{2}$" adhesive tape
Transparent dressing
Cotton
Sterile 2" x 2" gauze

➤ **PROCEDURE—Winged Catheter**

1. Insert the IV catheter according to "Peripheral Intravenous (IV) Cannulation" (Fig. 1-10).

   The piece of tape used to temporarily secure the catheter may be left in place if it does not cover the wings or insertion site.

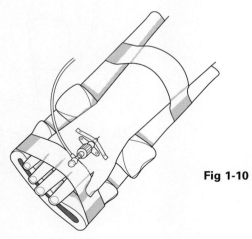

Fig 1-10

2. Place one piece of tape (1 cm x 10 cm) under the catheter hub, adhesive side up (Fig. 1-11).

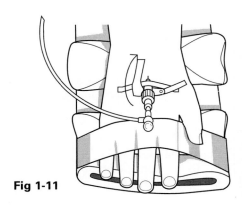

Fig 1-11

3. Fold the ends of tape over the wings of the catheter toward the child (Fig. 1-12).

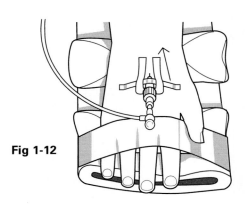

Fig 1-12

4. Place another piece of tape (1 cm x 5 cm) over the catheter hub. Keep the insertion site visible (Fig. 1-13).

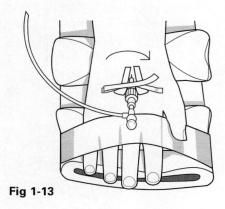

Fig 1-13

5. Cover with a transparent dressing (4 cm x 4 cm).[1,2] Do not cover the T-connector (Fig. 1-14).

   If a transparent dressing is not available, cover the site with a sterile 2" x 2" gauze pad.

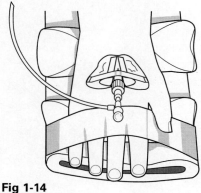

Fig 1-14

6. Place a small piece of cotton under the T-connector inject port (Fig. 1-15).

   Doing so will keep the catheter tip at the appropriate angle and away from the vein wall.[1]

7. Place a piece of tape (1 cm x 10 cm) over the inject port and tubing of the T-connector. Place the T-connector tubing beside the transparent dressing (Fig. 1-15).

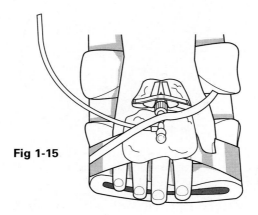

Fig 1-15

8. Secure the intravenous tubing approximately 10 cm from the insertion site with another piece of tape, 1 cm x 5 cm (Fig. 1-16).

9. Give the child positive feedback.

Fig 1-16

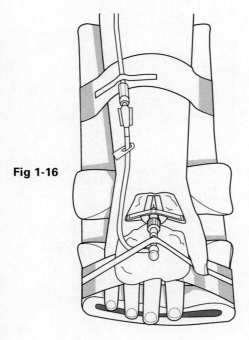

➤ *PROCEDURE—Non-Winged Catheter*

1. Insert the IV catheter according to "Peripheral Intravenous (IV) Cannulation" (Fig. 1-17).

   The piece of tape used to temporarily secure the catheter may be left in place if it does not cover the insertion site.

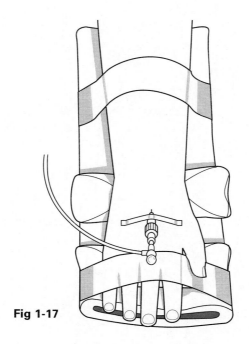

Fig 1-17

2. Place a piece of tape (1 cm x 10 cm) under the catheter hub, adhesive side up (Fig. 1-18).

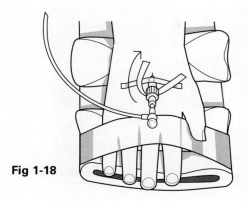

Fig 1-18

3. Cross the tape over the catheter hub toward the child[3] (Fig. 1-19).

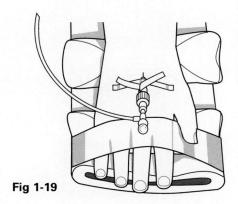

Fig 1-19

4. Place another piece of tape (1 cm x 5 cm) over the catheter hub. Keep the insertion site visible (Fig. 1-20).

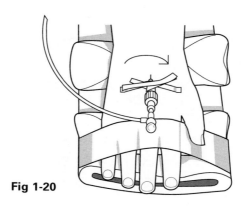

Fig 1-20

5. Continue with Steps 5 through 9 in the "Winged Catheter" section until the catheter is completely secured (Fig. 1-21).

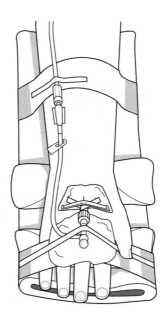

Fig 1-21

➤ *PROCEDURE—Scalp Catheter*

1. Insert the IV catheter according to "Peripheral Intravenous (IV) Cannulation."

   The piece of tape used to temporarily secure the catheter may be left in place if it does not cover the insertion site.

2. Follow Steps 1 through 4 in either the "Winged Catheter" or "Non-Winged Catheter" section.

3. To minimize the scalp area to be shaved, use a 2" x 2" gauze pad instead of a transparent dressing.

4. Place a medium-sized cotton ball under the T-connector, adjusting the cotton ball shape to the catheter.

   Doing so will stabilize the catheter tip in the vein, as well as the T-connector on the rounded surface of the scalp.

5. Wrap a piece of tape around the cotton ball (Fig. 1-22) and cross the ends over the T-connector and hub.

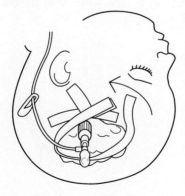

Fig 1-22

6. Place a piece of tape (1 cm x 10 cm) over the T-connector (Fig. 1-23).

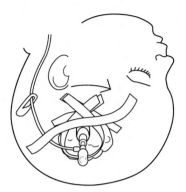

Fig 1-23

7. Cut a medicine cup in half lengthwise and pad the rough edges with gauze or tape. Cut a V in the bottom of the medicine cup (Fig. 1-24).

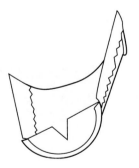

Fig 1-24

8. Turn the cup over the intravenous catheter and T-connector, with the T-connector inject hub fitting into the V.

Using the cup in this manner protects the catheter from dislodgement and may also be used for extremity IVs[1,2,3] (Fig. 1-25).

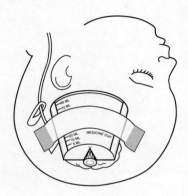

Fig 1-25

9. Give the child positive feedback.

References

[1]Wilson D: Neonatal IVs: practical tips, *Neonatal Netw* 11(2):49-53, 1992.

[2]Blatz S, Paes BA: Intravenous infusion by superficial vein in the neonate, *J Intraven Nurs* 13(2):122-128, 1990.

[3]Lynd M, Kesler RW, Bringelsen KA: Infusion procedures. In Lohr JA, ed.: *Pediatric outpatient procedures,* Philadelphia, 1991, JB Lippincott, pp. 275-287.

Intraosseous (IO) Needle Insertion

➤ **PURPOSE**

To rapidly identify appropriate sites and insertion techniques for IO needle placement.

➤ **SUPPLIES**

Bone marrow needle, spinal needle, or intraosseous needle
Nonsterile gloves
Povidone-iodine solution
IV extension tubing (2" to 3")
Three-way stopcock
60 ml syringe
IV infusion setup

➤ **PROCEDURE**

1. Determine the appropriateness for IO insertion.

Intraosseous access is recommended for rapid infusion of fluids and medications in children under 6 years of age.[2] Insertion is indicated in emergent situations in which effective ventilation is established and two attempts to establish peripheral venous access are unsuccessful or more than 90 seconds elapses. [1,2]

2. Set up IV infusion with extension tubing and a three-way stopcock (Fig. 1-26). Label bag and tubing with date and time infusion is begun.

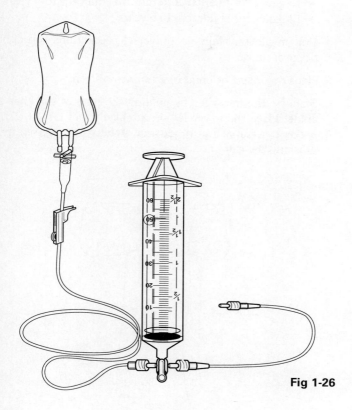

Fig 1-26

3. Assemble insertion equipment at bedside. Use the following list to determine appropriate size spinal or bone marrow needle:

- 18 gauge for infants less than three months
- 15 gauge for infants/ children three months to 5 years
- 13 gauge for children 5 to 6 years[3]

4. Put on gloves. Maintain universal precautions throughout the procedure.

5. Place the infant or child in a supine position.

6. Stabilize the lower leg by holding the limb at the knee and ankle. Place the lower leg on a folded towel (Fig. 1-27). To prevent personal injury, do not stabilize the extremity by grasping the calf.

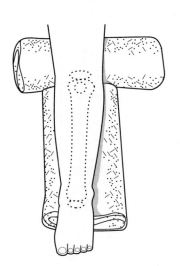

Fig 1-27

7. Select an appropriate site.

 • Tibial site: 1 to 3 cm below the tibial tuberosity (Fig. 1-28).

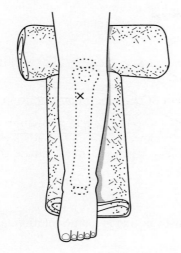

Fig 1-28

 • Distal femur site: 2 to 3 cm above the external condyles (Fig. 1-29).

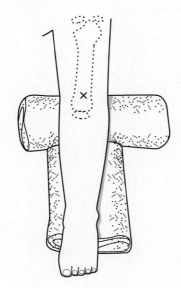

Fig 1-29

- Medial malleolus site: 1 to 3 cm proximal to the medial malleolus and posterior to the saphenous vein[4] (Fig. 1-30).

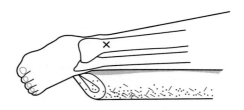

Fig 1-30

8. Cleanse site with povidone-iodine solution. Allow to dry for 60 seconds.

9. Insert the needle into the medial aspect of the tibia, approximately two fingerbreaths (1 to 3 cm) below the tibial tuberosity. Place the needle perpendicular or slightly inferior to the bone, which will prevent damage to the epiphyseal plate[1,2] (Fig. 1-31).

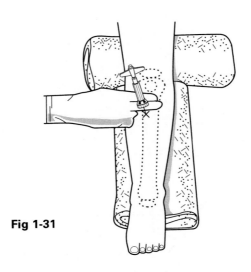

Fig 1-31

10. Advance the needle in a "screwing" motion until a "pop" is felt. The distance from the skin to the base of the needle is approximately 1 cm.[5] Remove stylet from needle if applicable.

11. Verify proper IO placement by one of the following methods:

   • Needle stands upright without support.[4]
   • Fluids flush easily without infiltration.
   • Blood or marrow particulate matter may be aspirated.

12. Attach extension tubing to the IO needle. Flush the needle, determine patency, and begin manual boluses using 60 ml syringe (see "Administering Intravenous [IV] Fluid Bolus.")

13. Secure the IO needle according to "Securing an Intraosseous (IO) Needle."

14. Document time of insertion, type and size of needle used, type of fluid or medications given, and amount of fluid (ml/kg) given.

15. Remove the IO needle following adequate fluid resuscitation and establishment of peripheral or central venous access.

References

[1]Chameides L: Vascular access. In Chameides L, ed.: *Textbook of pediatric advanced life support*, 1990, American Heart Association and American Academy of Pediatrics, pp. 37-46.

[2]Maloney-Harmon P: Initial assessment and stabilization of the critically injured child, *Crit Care Nurs Clin North Am* 3(3):399-409, 1991.

[3]Martin S: Procedures involving the cardiovascular system. In Bernardo LM, Bove M, eds.: *Pediatric emergency nursing procedures*, Boston, 1993, Jones and Bartlett, pp. 83-124.

[4]*Pediatric intraosseous infusions*, North Carolina EMS Training Program, Department of Human Resources.

[5]Scott M: Venous access in the field. In Hamilton J, Jacobs A, Morton D, eds.: *Pediatric trauma management for emergency medical services*, 1989, The Hemby Pediatric Trauma Institute.

Securing Intraosseous (IO) Needle

➤ **PURPOSE**

To adequately secure an IO needle and prevent it from being dislodged during short-term use of the needle.

➤ **SUPPLIES**

Nonsterile gauze
4" x 4" gauze pads
3" conforming gauze bandage or Kelly clamp
2" x 2" gauze pads
1/2" adhesive tape

➤ **PROCEDURE—*Winged Intraosseous Needle***

1. Put on gloves. Maintain universal precautions throughout the procedure.

2. Place folded 4" x 4" gauze pads on either side of the needle between the insertion point and the needle wings (Fig. 1-32).

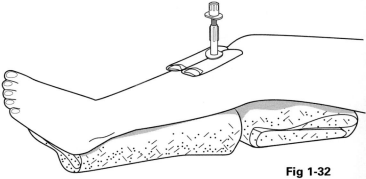

Fig 1-32

3. Using the rolled gauze, make a figure 8 around the calf and over the wings of the needle (Fig. 1-33).

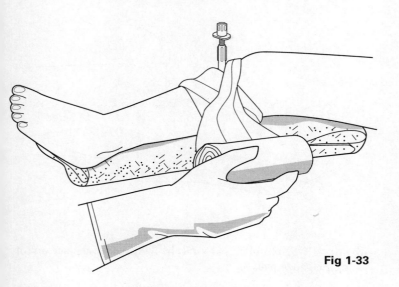

Fig 1-33

➤ *PROCEDURE—Non-Winged Intraosseous Needle*

1. Put on gloves. Maintain universal precautions throughout the procedure.

2. Place the 2" x 2" gauze pads on either side of the IO needle (Fig. 1-34).

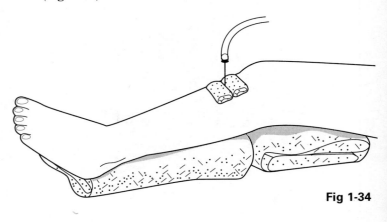

Fig 1-34

3. Attach the Kelly clamp around the IO needle and place on top of the gauze pads.

4. Place additional gauze pads between the skin and the body of the clamp if necessary (Fig. 1-35).

Fig 1-35

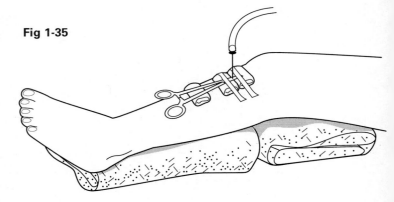

5. Place 3" pieces of tape across the clamp and the gauze pads to secure the clamp and needle in place.

Fluid and Medication Administration

Intravenous (IV) Fluid Bolus Administration

➤ **PURPOSE**

To quickly administer IV fluid boluses to an infant or child who requires volume resuscitation.

➤ **SUPPLIES**

60 ml syringe
IV infusion setup
Stopcock
IV extension set
Fluid
Nonsterile gloves

➤ **PROCEDURE**

1. Assemble supplies.

2. Wash hands.

3. Determine the appropriateness of the type and amount of fluid ordered.

   - **Isotonic fluids** (e.g., normal saline or lactated ringers) are the fluids of choice for volume resuscitation. Use 20 ml/kg for the initial bolus unless cardiogenic shock is suspected; if cardiogenic shock is suspected, administer 10 ml/kg.[1]
   - **Colloids** (e.g., 5% albumin, synthetic colloids, or packed red blood cells) may be ordered depending on the child's clinical condition. Use 10 ml/kg for the initial bolus with colloids. (To mix 5% albumin, see Box 1-1.)
   - **Glucose-containing solutions** (e.g., D_5W, $D_5^1/2NS$, $D_5^1/4NS$) are contraindicated since the induced hyperglycemia produces an osmotic diuresis.[1]

How to Mix 5% Albumin

1. Determine the amount of fluid ordered, e.g., 50 ml.
2. Divide the amount of fluid ordered by 5, e.g., $50 \div 5 = 10$ ml. This is the amount of 25% albumin needed. Once the vial of albumin is opened, it is stable for only 4 hours.[2]
3. Subtract this number from the total amount of fluid ordered, e.g., $50 - 10 = 40$ ml. This is the amount of diluent needed (LR or NS).*
4. Combine the 25% albumin (10 ml) and the diluent (40 ml) in a 60 ml syringe.

*The choice of LR or NS is dependent upon the child's clinical condition and the physician's preference.

4. Put on gloves. Maintain universal precautions throughout the procedure.

5. Assemble the IV infusion setup with a stopcock and IV extension set closest to the insertion site (Fig. 2-1). Attach the 60 ml syringe to the stopcock.

Fig 2-1

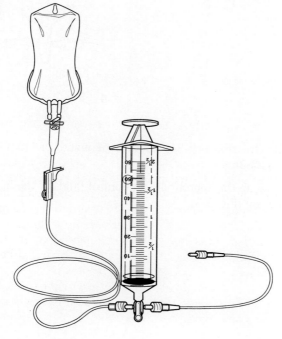

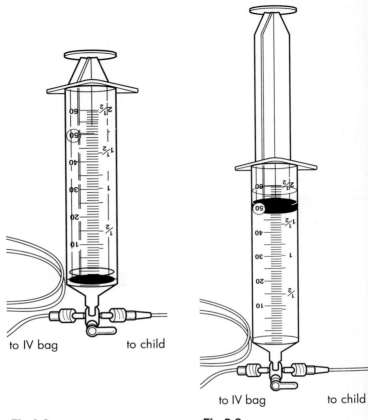

Fig 2-2   **Fig 2-3**

6. Turn the stopcock "off" to the patient and "on" to the IV fluid (Fig. 2-2).

7. Draw up the appropriate amount of fluid for the bolus from the bag (Fig. 2-3).

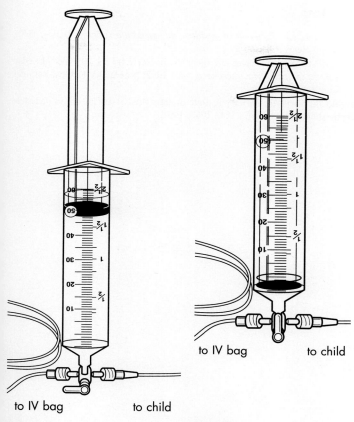

to IV bag   to child

Fig 2-4

to IV bag   to child

Fig 2-5

8. Turn the stopcock "off" to the IV fluid bag and "on" to the child (Fig. 2-4).

9. Deliver the bolus. Return the stopcock to the neutral position to avoid clotting the vein (Fig. 2-5).

10. Reassess the effectiveness of the fluid bolus and determine the need for another bolus.
    Rapid fluid resuscitation using volumes in excess of 60 ml/kg during the first hour is associated with improved outcome in children with septic shock.[3]

References

[1]Chamiedes L, ed.: *Textbook of pediatric advanced life support,* Dallas, 1988, American Heart Association.

[2]Norwood SS: Cardiovascular emergencies. In Norwood SS, Zaritsky AL, eds.: *Guidelines for pediatric emergency care,* 1992, Emergency Medical Services for Children Project.

[3]Carcillo JA, Davis AL, Zaritsky A: Role of early fluid resuscitation in pediatric septic shock, *JAMA* 266(9):1242-1245, 1991.

Calculating Maintenance Intravenous (IV) Fluid Requirements

➤ **PURPOSE**

To calculate maintenance IV fluid requirements based on weight for the critically ill or injured pediatric patient.

➤ **SUPPLIES**

Pencil or pen
Paper
Calculator
IV infusion pump
IV fluids
Pediatric emergency tape

➤ **PROCEDURE**

1. Assemble supplies.

2. Determine the child's weight in kilograms (kg). 1 kg = 2.2 lbs. *Use a pediatric emergency tape to estimate the child's weight based on his or her length if scales are not available.*

3. Calculate the child's daily or hourly maintenance fluid requirements based on the boxes on p. 50:[1]

   These calculations are for maintenance fluid requirements; children with specific diagnoses may require less fluid (e.g., children with cardiac, pulmonary, or renal failure or children with increased intracranial pressure).[1] Children in hypovolemic shock may require fluid boluses above their maintenance IV fluid requirement; boluses must be isotonic,

Body Weight	Formula for Daily Requirements
0-10 kg	100 ml/kg
11-20 kg	1000 ml for first 10 kg plus 50 ml/kg for every kg over 10 kg
21-30 kg	1500 ml for first 20 kg plus 25 ml/kg for every kg over 20 kg

From Hazinski MF: *Nursing care of the critically ill child*, ed 2, St. Louis, 1992, Mosby.

Body Weight	Formula for Hourly Requirements
0-10 kg	4 ml/kg/hour
11-20 kg	40 ml/hour for first 10 kg plus 2 ml/kg/hour for every kg over 10 kg
21-30 kg	60 ml/hour for first 20 kg plus 1 ml/kg/hour for every kg over 20 kg

From Hazinski MF: *Nursing care of the critically ill child*, ed 2, St. Louis, 1992, Mosby.

non–glucose-containing solutions (see "Intravenous (IV) Fluid Bolus Administration").

4. Administer recommended maintenance fluids:[2]

   • $D_5^1/4NS$ for infants and children
   • $D_{10}^1/4NS$ for newborns
   Potassium may be added after urine output is established.

5. Use an infusion pump to administer the IV fluids. To ensure safety, set the total pump volume to be delivered for a volume equal to two hours of the child's hourly fluid requirement.

References

[1]Hazinski MF: *Nursing care of the critically ill child,* ed 2, St. Louis, 1992, Mosby.

[2]Johnson KB: *The Harriet Lane handbook,* ed 13, St. Louis, 1993, Mosby, p. 164.

Calculating Pediatric Doses

➤ **PURPOSE**

To correctly calculate pediatric doses based on weight or body surface area (BSA).

➤ **SUPPLIES**

Pen or pencil
Paper
Calculator
Pediatric pharmacology reference manual:

- Benitz WE, Tatro DS: *The pediatric drug handbook,* ed 2, Chicago, 1988, Mosby.
- Johnson KB: *The Harriet Lane handbook,* ed 13, St. Louis, 1993, Mosby.

Pediatric emergency tape
Medication ordered

➤ **PROCEDURE**

1. Assemble supplies.

2. Compare the medication administration record with the original written order to ensure the order was transcribed correctly.
   If the order is ambiguous or the handwriting is difficult to decipher, consult with the physician to clarify. Medication orders must be written in "mg," not "cc" or "ml." Request the physician to rewrite the order clearly and/or print the order. Errors in transcription and misinterpretation are common.[1,2]

3. Determine the child's weight in kilograms (kg). 1 kg = 2.2 lbs. Or calculate using a BSA nomogram from a general pediatric text (e.g., Vaughan VC, Behrman RE, eds.: *Nelson textbook of pediatrics,* Philadelphia, 1975, WB Saunders).

   Unless the child is unusually tall, short, thin, or overweight, there are minor differences between calculations according to weight as compared to calculations according to BSA.[3] Generally, pediatric dose recommendations are based on weight, i.e. mg/kg.

4. Determine the recommended dose range for the child's weight, age, and disease process by consulting a pediatric pharmacology reference manual. This dose is usually expressed in "mg/kg/day".

   EXAMPLE:
   Cefoxitin recommended dose for infants and children = 80-160 mg/kg/day divided by Q4-6hr

   If the recommended dose is expressed as "mg/kg/dose," see Step 7.

5. Calculate the child's recommended dose range (safe and effective) per day by multiplying the child's weight (in kg) by the recommended milligrams.[3]

   EXAMPLE:
   Child's weight = 4 kg

   Cefoxitin = 80-160 mg/kg/day divided by Q4-6hr

   4 kg × 160 mg = 640 mg/day = recommended safe dose for this child

   4 kg × 80 mg = 320 mg/day = recommended effective dose for this child

6. Multiply the ordered dose by the dose frequency to calculate the ordered total daily dose.

   EXAMPLE:
   Order reads "Cefoxitin 125 mg IV Q6hr"

   125 mg × 4 (number of times given in 24 hours period) = total daily dose of 500 mg

   Compare the ordered total daily dose with the recommended total daily dose range. If the dose ordered is incorrect, con-

sult with the physician. If the physician acknowledges the medication dose as conflicting with the recommended dose and explains the reasoning for the dose, document on the medication administration record that the physician was consulted and the dose verified.

7. If the recommended dose is listed as "mg/kg/dose," multiply the child's weight by the recommended dose and compare your calculated dose with the dose ordered. Also compare the time interval ordered with the time interval recommended.

    This step is particularly important for medications recommended as "mg/kg/dose," as too frequent or infrequent intervals will have a dramatic effect on the total amount of medication the child receives. If the ordered dose or interval is incorrect, consult with the physician. If the physician acknowledges the medication dose as conflicting with the recommended dose and explains the reasoning for the dose, document on the medication administration record that the physician was consulted and the dose verified.

8. Confirm calculations with a colleague if the medication ordered is digoxin, insulin, aminophylline, potassium, a narcotic, or if you have questions regarding your calculation.

    Errors in calculation and administration of incorrect doses account for as many as 32% to 43% of all medication errors.[1,4]

9. Use precalculated drug sheets based on the child's weight[5,6,7,8] (Fig. 2-6) or the pediatric emergency tape for code drug doses. Place the drug sheet at the child's bedside on admission.

Fig 2-6

Service _____ Attending _____ Resident _____

Name _____ DOB _____ Weight ____kg Date _____
ETT Size_____ Taped at _____ Trach Size _____
Allergies _____

EMERGENCY DRUG CALCULATIONS FOR CHILDREN

Drug (concentration)	Dose in mg	Dose in ml
Epinephrine 1:10,000 (0.1 mg/ml)	0.01 mg/kg=_____mg	0.1 ml/kg = _____ml
Epinephrine 1:1000 (1.0 mg/ml)	0.1 mg/kg = _____mg	0.1 ml/kg = _____ml
Atropine (0.1 mg/ml)	0.02 mg/kg = _____mg (maximum dose = 0.5 mg, minumum dose = 0.1 mg)	0.2 ml/kg = _____ml
CaCl$_2$ 10% (100 mg/ml)	20mg/kg = _____mg	0.2 ml/kg = _____ml
Adenosine (3 mg/ml)	0.1 mg/kg = _____mg	0.03 ml/kg = _____ml
Dextrose 25% (25g/100ml) (dilute D$_{50}$ 1:1 with sterile H$_2$O)	0.5 g/kg = _____gm (up to 1 g/kg)	2 ml/kg of D$_{25}$ = _____m
Na bicarb (1 mEq/ml) (dilute 1:1 with saline)	1 mEq/kg = _____mEq	1ml/kg = _____ml
Naloxone (1 mg/ml)	0.1 mg/kg = _____mg	0.1ml/kg = _____ml
Lorazepam (4 mg/ml)	0.1 mg/kg = _____mg	0.025 ml/kg = _____ml
Diazepam (5 mg/ml)	0.2 mg/kg = _____mg (slow IV push, undiluted up to 0.4 mg/kg/dose)	0.04 ml/kg = _____ml
Defibrillation	2 joules/kg = _____joules	

References

[1]Vincer MJ et al: Drug errors and incidents in a neonatal intensive care unit, *Am J Dis Child* 143(6):737-740, 1989.

[2]Rudy C: A drop or a dropper: the risk of overdose, *J Pediatr Health Care* 6(1):40, 51-52, 1992.

[3]Wink DM: Giving infants and children drugs: precision = caution = safety, *MCN Am J Matern Child Nurse* 16(6):317-321, 1991.

[4]Raju TNK et al: Medication errors in neonatal and pediatric intensive-care units, *Lancet* 2(8659):374-376, 1989.

[5]Briggs L, Beyda D: Giving pediatric code drugs, *Nursing* 16(7):56, 1986.

[6]Hazinski MF: Reducing calculation errors in drug dosages: the pediatric critical information sheet, *Pediatr Nurs* 12(2):138-140, 1986.

[7]Fonner CJ, Rushton CH, Fletcher AB: Preparation for neonatal emergencies: a neonatal emergency medication sheet, *Pediatr Nurs* 15(5):527-529, 1989.

[8]Rockney RM, Alario AJ, Lewander WJ: Revised pediatric dose card, *Am J Dis Child* 144(3):272-274, 1990.

Intravenous (IV) Retrograde Delivery

➤ **PURPOSE**

To safely administer IV medications over a period of time by retrograde delivery.

➤ **SUPPLIES**

Nonsterile gloves
Commercially available retrograde set **or**
Connecting IV tubing with an injection port at each end or a stopcock at each end
Two 10 ml syringes (with needles attached if using injection ports instead of stopcocks)
One 3 ml syringe
Alcohol swabs
Normal saline
Medication ordered

➤ **PROCEDURE**

1. Determine the appropriateness of retrograde delivery for the medication ordered.
   Situations where retrograde medication delivery may be appropriate include:

   • *antibiotics given over 10 to 30 minutes*
   • *patients whose total fluid restrictions cannot accommodate additional medication fluid volume*

   Situations where retrograde medication delivery is not appropriate include:

- *IV push medications*
- *medications diluted in large volume (> 10 ml)*
- *medications given over 30 minutes or longer, e.g. vancomycin, amphotericin*
- *in conjunction with lipid,[1] aminophylline, insulin, or cardiotonic infusions[2]*
- *medications that require drug levels following this dose*

Retrograde delivery inconsistencies may influence peak serum concentration levels;[3] the most reliable and consistent method of IV medication infusion recommended is a small volume pump and a separate heparin lock.[1,3] If either of these are not available and the drug must be given over time, institute the retrograde delivery system.

2. Assemble supplies.

3. Wash hands.

4. Draw up medicine in a 10 ml syringe and dilute according to the pharmaceutical package insert.
   If your institution's pharmacy mixes the medication, ensure that it has been diluted also.

5. Determine the maximum amount of fluid the IV connecting tubing holds. (This is often listed on the package.) To avoid displacing medication along with maintenance fluid, the medication volume should not exceed 50% of the volume of the connecting tubing.[3]

   EXAMPLE:
   If the volume of the connecting tubing or retrograde set is 6 ml, the medication volume should not exceed 3 ml.

6. Determine the potential infusion rate of the medication placed in the continuous infusion line.

   EXAMPLE:

   $$\frac{4\ ml - (volume\ of\ medication\ in\ ml)}{20\ minutes - (time\ in\ minutes)} = \frac{12\ ml - (hourly\ ml\ delivered\ by\ IV)}{60\ minutes - (minutes\ in\ an\ hour)}$$

   Ascertain if the result is an appropriate time frame for the medication to be delivered, or if the maintenance fluid rate can be adjusted.

7. Explain procedure to parents and, if appropriate, to the child.

8. Put on gloves. Maintain universal precautions throughout the procedure.

9. If using two stopcocks, place an empty 10 ml syringe at stopcock 2 (Fig. 2-7). If using two injection ports, swab both ports with alcohol and place an empty 10 ml syringe at the injection port furthest from the child.

Fig 2-7

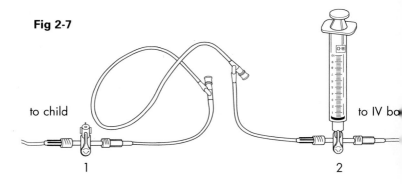

to child   to IV bag

1   2

10. Draw up 1 ml of NS in a 3 ml syringe.
    This is used to provide a barrier between the medication and the maintenance fluid. If the medication is compatible with the maintenance fluid, go to Step 14.

11. Attach the syringe with 1 ml NS to stopcock 1 (or inject in port). Turn the stopcock off (or clamp the IV tubing) to the IV bag and inject 0.5 ml of NS (Fig. 2-8).
    This forces the fluid to move toward the child and is the first half of the barrier.

Fig 2-8

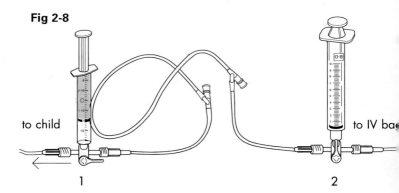

to child   to IV bag

1   2

12. Turn stopcock 2 (or clamp the IV tubing) off to the IV bag.

13. Turn stopcock 1 off (or clamp the IV tubing) to the child and inject the remaining 0.5 ml of NS (Fig. 2-9).
This forces the fluid to move away from the child and completes the barrier.

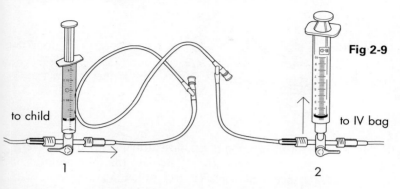

Fig 2-9

to child

to IV bag

1   2

14. Keep stopcock 1 off (or the IV tubing clamped) to the child and place syringe with diluted medicine in stopcock 1. Keep stopcock 2 off to the IV bag. Slowly inject the medicine; the medicine is forced to move away from the child (retrograde) and is sandwiched between the NS barrier. The maintenance fluid in the tubing is displaced into the empty syringe distally (Fig. 2-10).[1]

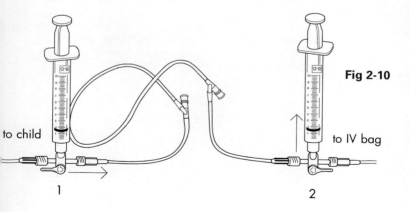

Fig 2-10

to child

to IV bag

1   2

15. Turn the stopcock to neutral (or unclamp tubing) and remove syringes (Fig. 2-11).

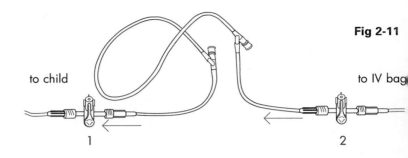

Fig 2-11

to child

to IV bag

1

2

16. Document medication given, dose, time, method of delivery, and your initials/signature. Calculate the total amount of maintenance fluid displaced over 24 hours and consult with physician regarding the need for replacement of glucose or nutrients.[1,2,4]

References

[1]Hargrove C: Administration of IV medication in the NICU: the development of a procedure, *Neonatal Netw* 6(2):41-49, 1987.

[2]Axton SE, Fugate T: A protocol for pediatric IV meds, *Am J Nurs* 87(7):943-945, 1987.

[3]Nahata MC: Influence of infusion methods on therapeutic drug monitoring in pediatric patients, *Drug Intell Clin Pharm* 20(5):367-369, 1986.

[4]Burch SM, Chadwick JR: Use of a retroset in the delivery of intravenous medications in the neonate, *Neonatal Netw* 6(2):51-54, 1987.

Calculating Inotropic Infusions

➤ **PURPOSE**

To calculate inotropic infusion dosages correctly and to prepare the infusion for the critically ill or injured pediatric patient.

➤ **SUPPLIES**

Pen or pencil
Paper
Calculator
Pediatric emergency tape
Infusion pump
IV infusion pump tubing
500 ml bag of D_5W
IV buretrol
Medication ordered

➤ **PROCEDURE**

1. Assemble supplies.

2. Determine the child's weight in kilograms (kg). 1 kg = 2.2 lbs. *Use a pediatric emergency tape to estimate the child's weight based on his or her length if scales are not available.*

3. Wash hands.

4. Close the roller clamp above the buretrol and spike the bag of D_5W with the IV buretrol.

5. Place the IV bag and buretrol on an IV pole or some other stationary hook. Close the roller clamp below the buretrol and open the roller clamp above the buretrol. Allow 20 to 30 ml of D₅W to fill the buretrol and then close the roller clamp above the buretrol (Fig. 2-12).
Do not allow the D₅W to purge the line.

Fig 2-12

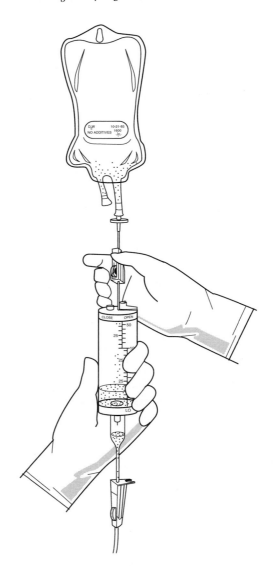

6. Calculate the amount of medication to add according to the "rule of sixes."[1]

- For *epinephrine, norepinephrine, isoproterenol,* and *prostaglandin E_1,* multiply the child's weight (kg) by 0.6. The product is the number of milligrams of medication to add to the buretrol to total 100 ml.
  Then 1 ml/hr = 0.1 µg/kg/minute.

- For *dopamine, dobutamine, nitroprusside,* and *nitroglycerin,* multiply the child's weight (kg) by 6. The product is the number of milligrams of medication to add to the buretrol to total 100 ml.
  Then 1 ml/hr = 1 µg/kg/ minute.

- For *lidocaine* multiply the child's weight (kg) by 60. The product is the number of milligrams of medication to add to the buretrol to total 100 ml.
  Then 1 ml/hr = 10 µg/kg/minute.

NOTE: *The "rule of sixes" may not work well for children over 20 kg. For larger children, use a more dilute solution (i.e., a 1:10 dilution).*

EXAMPLE:
Child's weight = 30 kg

To make an epinephrine drip:
- *30 kg × 0.6 = 18 mg to add to the buretrol to total 100 ml Then 1 ml/hr = 0.1 µg/kg/min.*
Instead, use a 1:10 dilution:
- *30 kg × 0.06 = 1.8 mg to add to the buretrol to total 100 ml. Then 10 ml/hr = 0.1 µg/kg/min.*

7. Confirm the calculation with a colleague.
Errors in calculations and administering incorrect doses account for as many as 32% to 43% of all medication errors.[3,4]

8. Add the medication to the buretrol (Fig. 2-13) and then fill the buretrol to the 100 ml marker with D_5W. Gently agitate the solution.

Fig 2-13

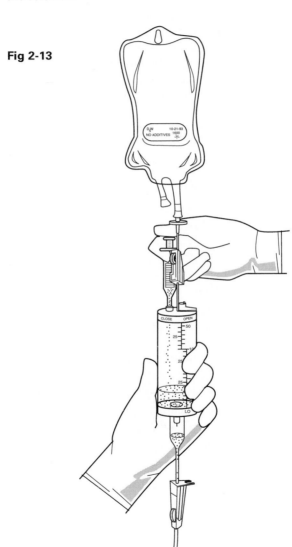

9. Place a colored sticker or plastic clamp between the bag of
   D$_5$W and the buretrol; this serves as a reminder that fluid
   from the bag cannot be added to the buretrol without further
   medication (Fig. 2-14).

Fig 2-14

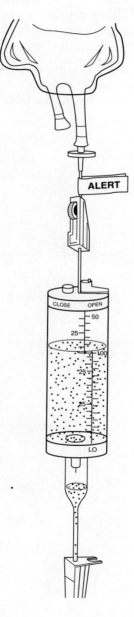

10. Purge the IV tubing with the medication-filled fluid.
    This is to guarantee that when the tubing is connected to the patient, the fluid in the tubing nearest the patient contains the inotrope.

11. Use an infusion pump for administration of the inotrope. Label the pump with the inotrope and the concentration, i.e., "1 ml/hr = 0.1 µg/kg/minute Epinephrine."

12. Place the inotrope infusion at the port closest to the patient. If the infusion is running at a slow rate, place a maintenance intravenous fluid line behind the inotrope.

13. Label the buretrol with the date, time, child's name, weight, amount of medication added, concentration, and your initials (Figs. 2-15 and 2-16).

14. Document the time the infusion was started, the child's response, and the titrated level.

Fig 2-15

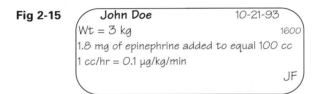

John Doe   10-21-93
Wt = 3 kg   1600
1.8 mg of epinephrine added to equal 100 cc
1 cc/hr = 0.1 µg/kg/min
                                    JF

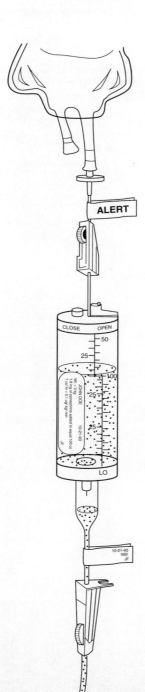

Fig 2-16

References

[1]Hazinski MF: Cardiovascular disorders. In Hazinski MF, ed.: *Nursing care of the critically ill child*, ed 2, St. Louis, 1992, Mosby, p. 117-395.

[2]Norwood SS: Vascular access, fluids and medication administration. In Norwood SS, Zaritsky AL, eds.: *Guidelines for pediatric emergency care*, 1992, Emergency Medical Services for Children Project.

[3]Vincer MJ et al: Drug errors and incidents in a neonatal intensive care unit, *Am J Dis Child* 143(6):737-740, 1989.

[4]Raju TNK et al: Medication errors in neonatal and pediatric intensive care units, *Lancet* 2(8659):374-376, 1989.

Table 2-1	Pediatric Intravenous Administration				
Generic Name (Brand Name)	Initial Concentration	Maximum Concentration for Peripheral IV Administration	Recommended Infusion Time	Minimum Infusion Time	Compatible IV Solutions
Acetazolamide (Diamox)	100 mg/ml	100 mg/ml	100 mg/min	100 mg/min	Any dextrose-saline solutions, LR
Acyclovir Sodium (Zorivax)	50 mg/ml	7 mg/ml	60 min	60 min	Any dextrose-saline solutions, LR
Albumin	5% = 50 mg/ml 25% = 250 mg/ml		5%: Do not exceed 2-4 ml/min 25%: Do not exceed 1 ml/min	5%: Do not exceed 2-4 ml/min 25%: Do not exceed 1 ml/min	NS preferred; compatible in D_5W, $D_{10}W$
Amikacin (Amikin)	250 mg/ml	5 mg/ml	30-60 min; infants, 1-2 hrs	30-60 min; infants, 1-2 hrs	Any dextrose-saline solutions, LR
Aminophylline	25 mg/ml	25 mg/ml	20-30 min	not > 25 mg/min	Any dextrose-saline solutions, LR
Amphotericin B (Fungizone)	5 mg/ml	0.1 mg/ml	over 6 hrs	over 4 hrs	D_5W
Ampicillin (Omnipen Polycillin)	Add 10 ml NS to 1 Gm vial for concentration of 100 mg/ml	30 mg/ml	15 min	100 mg/min	Most stable in NS; can use dextrose solutions, but not in high concentrations

Continued.

Table 2-1	Pediatric Intravenous Administration—cont'd				
Generic Name (Brand Name)	Initial Concentration	Maximum Concentration for Peripheral IV Administration	Recommended Infusion Time	Minimum Infusion Time	Compatible IV Solutions
Ampicillin/ Sulbactam (Unasyn)	Add 9.2 ml of NS to 1.5 Gm vial for concentration of 100 mg/ml ampicillin	30 mg/ml ampicillin	15-30 min	15 min	NS preferred; also compatible in dextrose containing solutions, LR
Azlocillin (Azlin)	100 mg/ml	100 mg/ml	20-50 min	5 min	Any dextrose-saline solution, LR
Aztreonam (Azactam)	200 mg/ml	20 mg/ml	20-60 min	3-5 min	Any dextrose-saline solution, LR
Calcium Chloride	100 mg/ml	20 mg/ml	30 min	100 mg/min	Any dextrose-saline solution
Calcium Gluconate	100 mg/ml	20 mg/ml	30 min	100 mg/min	Any dextrose-saline solution, LR
Cefazolin (Ancef, Kefzol)	100 mg/ml	100 mg/ml	15 min	3-5 min	Any dextrose-saline solution, LR
Cefotaxime (Claforan)	100 mg/ml	100 mg/ml	10-30 min	3-5 min	Any dextrose-saline solution, LR
Cefoxitin (Mefoxitin)	100 mg/ml	100 mg/ml	20-60 min	3-5 min	Any dextrose-saline solution, LR
Ceftazidine (Fortaz, Tazidime)	100 mg/ml	100 mg/ml	10-30 min	3-5 min	Any dextrose-saline solution, LR

Drug					
Ceftriaxone (Rocephin)	100 mg/ml	40 mg/ml	10-30 min	3-5 min	Any dextrose-saline solution
Cefuroxime (Zinacef)	100 mg/ml	50-100 mg/ml	15-60 min	3-5 min	Any dextrose-saline solution
Chloramphenicol Sodium Succinate (Chloromycetin)	100 mg/ml	100 mg/ml	30-60 min	100 mg/min	Any dextrose-saline solution, LR
Chlorpromazine (Thorazine)	25 mg/ml	1 mg/ml	0.5 mg/min	0.5 mg/min	NS preferred; also compatible in dextrose solutions, LR
Cimetidine (Tagamet)	150 mg/ml	15 mg/ml	15-30 min	2-5 min	Any dextrose-saline solutions; LR
Clindamycin Phosphate (Cleocin)	150 mg/ml	12 mg/ml	30-60 min	10 min not > 30 mg/min	Any dextrose-saline solution, LR
Cyclosporine (Sandimmune)	50 mg/ml	2.5 mg/ml	2-6 hrs	2 hrs	D5W, NS
Dexamethasone (Decadron)	4 mg/ml	4 mg/ml	10-20 min	1-5 min	Any dextrose-saline solution
Diazepam (Valium)	5 mg/ml	Do not dilute	3 min Not > 5 mg/min	not > 5 mg/min	Not recommended
Diazomide (Hyperstat)	15 mg/ml	Do not dilute	15-30 sec	rapid IV injection preferred	Not recommended

Continued.

Table 2-1	Pediatric Intravenous Administration				
Generic Name (Brand Name)	Initial Concentration	Maximum Concentration for Peripheral IV Administration	Recommended Infusion Time	Minimum Infusion Time	Compatible IV Solutions
Digoxin (Lanoxin)	100 µg/ml 250 µg/ml	250 µg/ml	5-15 min	5 min	D$_5$W, NS
Diphenhydramine (Benadryl)	50 mg/ml	30 mg/ml	over 15 min	5 min not > 25 mg/min	Any dextrose-saline solution
Erythromycin	50 mg/ml	5 mg/ml	60 min	20-60 min	Any dextrose-saline solution
Ethacrynic Acid (Edecrin)	1 mg/ml	1 mg/ml	20-30 min	5-10 min	Any dextrose-saline solution
Furosemide (Lasix)	10 mg/ml	10 mg/ml	over 10 min	1-2 min not > 4 mg/min or 0.5 mg/kg/min	Any dextrose-saline solution
Gentamicin (Garamycin)	10 mg/ml 40 mg/ml	40 mg/ml	30-60 min; infants, 1-2 hrs	30 min	Any dextrose-saline solution
Hydralazine (Apresoline)	20 mg/ml	20 mg/ml	0.2 mg/kg/min	do not exceed 0.2 mg/kg/min	Any dextrose-saline solution
Hydrocortisone Sodium Phosphate (Hydrocortone) **Sodium Succinate** (Solu-cortef)	50 mg/ml	50 mg/ml	over 30 min	slow IVP over 30 sec for doses < 100 mg; over 10 min for doses > 500 mg	Any dextrose-saline solution

Imipenem-Cilistatin (Primaxin)	50 mg/ml		over 40-60 min for doses>1 Gm	over 20-30 min for doses < 500 mg	NS preferred
Labetalol (Normodyne, Trandate)	5 mg/ml	Dilute in convenient volume	over 2 min	not faster than 2 mg/min	Any dextrose-saline solution, LR
Lorazepam (Ativan)	2 mg/ml	1 mg/ml	2 min	not > 2 mg/min	D5W preferred, also compatible with NS
Magnesium Sulfate	500 mg/ml	100 mg/ml	3 hrs	do not exceed 125 mg/kg/hr	Any dextrose-saline solution
Mannitol	20% = 200 mg/ml 25% = 250 mg/ml	250 mg/ml	30-60 min	3-5 min	Usually not diluted
Methyl-Prednisolone (Solu-medrol)	40 mg/ml 62.5 mg/ml	40 mg/ml	20-30 min	2-3 min; for doses > 500 mg give over 15-20 min	Any dextrose-saline solution
Metoclopramide (Reglan)	5 mg/ml	5 mg/ml	>10 mg over 15 min	< 10 mg over 1-2 min	Any dextrose-saline solution
Metronidazole (Flagyl R.T.U.)	5 mg/ml	No dilution needed	60 min	60 min	Any dextrose-saline solution
Mezlocillin (Mezlin)	100 mg/ml	100 mg/ml	30 min	3-5 min	Any dextrose-saline solution
Midazolam (Versed)	1 mg/ml 5 mg/ml	5 mg/ml	2 min	2 min	D5W, NS, LR

Continued.

Table 2-1	Pediatric Intravenous Administration—cont'd				
Generic Name (Brand Name)	Initial Concentration	Maximum Concentration for Peripheral IV Administration	Recommended Infusion Time	Minimum Infusion Time	Compatible IV Solutions
Morphine Sulphate	1 mg/ml 2 mg/ml 5 mg/ml 10 mg/ml 15 mg/ml	5 mg/ml	3-5 min	3-5 min	Any dextrose-saline solution
Nafcillin (Nafcil, Unipen)	100 mg/ml	40 mg/ml	15-30 min	5-10 min	Any dextrose-saline solution
Naloxone (Narcan)	1 mg/ml		< 30 sec	< 30 sec	D$_5$W, NS
Oxacillin (Bactocill)	100 mg/ml	100 mg/ml	15-30 min	100 mg/min	Any dextrose-saline solution
Penicillan G Potassium	100,000 units/ml	100,000 U/ml	15-60 min	15-30 min	Any dextrose-saline solution
Penicillan G Sodium	500,000 units/ml	100,000 U/ml	15-60 min	15-30 min	Any dextrose-saline solution
Pentobarbital (Nembutal)	50 mg/ml	50 mg/ml	10 min	1-2 mg/kg over 3-5 min	Any dextrose-saline solution
Phenobarbital	20 mg/ml 30 mg/ml 130 mg/ml	Do not dilute	3-5 min not 1 >mg/kg/min	not > 1 mg/kg/min	Any dextrose-saline solution

Drug					
Phenytoin Sodium (Dilantin)	50 mg/ml	Do not dilute	0.5 mg/kg/min	not >1 mg/kg/min	NS
Phytoadione (Vt.K) (Aquamephyton)	10 mg/ml	10 mg/ml	15 min	not > 1 mg/min	Any dextrose-saline solution
Piperacillin (Pipracil)	200 mg/ml	200 mg/ml	30 min	3-5 min	Any dextrose-saline solution, LR
Prednisolone (Hydeltrasol)	20 mg/ml		1-3 min	1-3 min	Any dextrose-saline solution
Promethazine (Phenergan)	25 mg/ml	25 mg/ml	25 mg/min	25 mg/min	Any dextrose-saline solution
Propranolol (Inderal)	1 mg/ml	Do not dilute	10 min	not > 1 mg/min	Do not dilute
Rantidine (Zantac)	25 mg/ml	2.5 mg/ml	15-20 min	5 min	Any dextrose-saline solution
Sodium Bicarbonate	1 mEq/ml 0.5 mEq/ml	0.5 mEq/ml for children < 2 yrs; 1 m Eq/ml for children > 2 yrs		1-3 mEq/kg over 1-2 min; not 10 mEq/min	Any dextrose-saline solution
Ticarcillan (Ticar)	250 mg/ml	50 mg/ml	30 min	100 mg/min	Any dextrose-saline solution, LR
Ticarcillin/ Clavulanate (Timentin)	200 mg/ml as ticarcillin	50 mg/ml as ticarcillin	30 min	30 min	D5W, NS, LR
Tobramycin (Nebcin)	10 mg/ml 40 mg/ml	40 mg/ml	30-60 min	30 min	D_5W, NS, LR

Continued.

Table 2-1	Pediatric Intravenous Administration—cont'd				
Generic Name (Brand Name)	Initial Concentration	Maximum Concentration for Peripheral IV Administration	Recommended Infusion Time	Minimum Infusion Time	Compatible IV Solutions
Trimethoprim Sulfamethoxazole (Bactrim, Septraz, TMP-SMX)	16 mg/ml TMP 80 mg/ml SMX	1 ml/15 ml	60-90 min	60 min	D5W only
Vancomycin (Vancomycin)	50 mg/ml	5 mg/ml	60 min	60 min	Any dextrose-saline solution, LR

Sources:

Fiacco L et al: *Administration guidelines for intravenous medication in pediatric patients,* 1991, University of North Carolina Pediatric Pharmacy Protocol.

Taketomo CK, Hodding JH, Kraus DM: *1993-94 pediatric dosage handbook,* ed 2, Hudson, Ohio, 1993, Lexi-Comp Inc.

Aggour T, Osake J: *Pharmacy Practice News* Nov 1991, pp. 10-12.

Gura KM: Parenteral drug administration guidelines for the pediatric patient: one hospital's recommendations, *Hospital Pharmacy* 28(3): 221-223, 227-228, 231-236, 239-242, 1993.

CHAPTER

3

Oxygenation and Ventilation

Administration of Oxygen (O_2)

➤ **PURPOSE**

To provide supplemental O_2 by the appropriate method to a pediatric patient whose clinical presentation indicates respiratory distress.

➤ **SUPPLIES**

O_2 delivery device
O_2 connecting tubing
Flow meter
O_2 source

➤ **PROCEDURE**

1. Determine the need for oxygen administration.
   Oxygen deficiency in the pediatric patient can ultimately lead to respiratory failure and cardiopulmonary arrest.[1] The goal of therapy is to restore and maintain O_2 delivery to the cells.[2]

2. Identify the appropriate method of O_2 administration for the infant or child (see Tables 3-1 and 3-2).
   Choose an oxygen delivery system that is appropriate for the child's age and needs. Ultimately it is the child's minute ventilation that will determine the oxygen concentration delivered, and the following guidelines may need to be modified on an individual basis.[2,3]

Table 3-1 Methods to Provide Maximum Oxygenation by Age

Age	Method
Neonates and infants	Oxygen hood
Infants and small toddlers	Nasal cannula, blow-by, face mask
Toddlers and preschoolers	Nasal cannula, blow-by, face mask
School-age children and adolescents	Non-rebreathing mask

From Aoki BY, McCloskey K: *Evaluation, stabilization, and transport of the critically ill child,* St Louis, 1992, Mosby, pp. 1-16.

Table 3-2 Flow Rates of Oxygen Delivery Systems

Oxygen Delivery Systems	Flow Rate	Maximum O_2 Delivery
Blow-by	6 L/min	80%
Oxygen hood	10-15 L/min	100%
Nasal cannula	1-6 L/min	44%
Simple mask	6-10 L/min	60%
Partial rebreather mask	10-12 L/min	60%
Non-rebreather mask	10-12 L/min	95%

From Chameides L: Airway management. In Chameides L, ed: *Textbook of pediatric advanced life support,* 1990, American Heart Association and American Academy of Pediatrics; Norwood SS: Respiratory emergencies. In Norwood SS, Zaritsky AL, eds: *Guidelines to pediatric emergency care,* 1992, Emergency Medical Services for Children Project; and Rowe PC, ed: *The Harriet Lane handbook,* Chicago, 1987, Year Book.

3. Assemble equipment at the child's bedside. Test oxygen source for effectiveness and determine the O_2 supply.

4. Attach O_2 tubing to O_2 source and connect to the delivery device.

5. Explain to the child and the family the need for oxygen administration and how the device will work (e.g., "the face mask will be placed over your nose and mouth"). Explain to the child how the oxygen delivery device will feel and the need for the device to stay in place.

6. Place the chosen device on the child.
On an infant or toddler it may be necessary to tape the nasal cannula to the cheeks to prevent displacement.

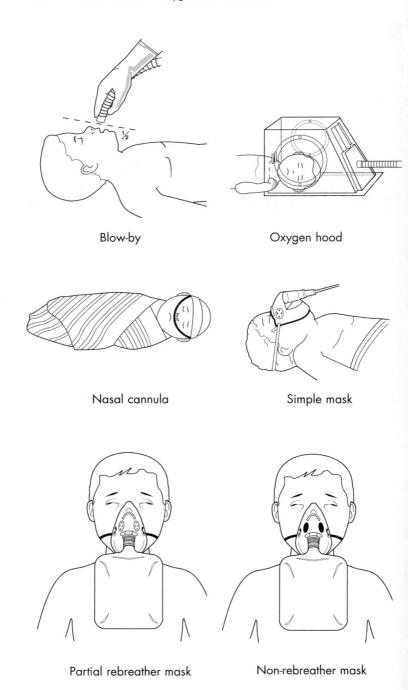

Blow-by

Oxygen hood

Nasal cannula

Simple mask

Partial rebreather mask

Non-rebreather mask

7. Give the child positive feedback.

8. Document the method of oxygenation, flow rate, time therapy was initiated, and how the child responded to therapy.

9. Use arterial or capillary blood gases and /or pulse oximetry to monitor the effectiveness of oxygen therapy[2] (Fig. 3-1).

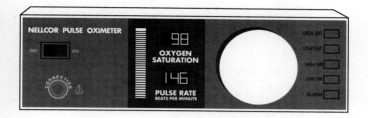

Fig 3-1

References

[1]Chameides L: Airway management. In Chameides L, ed.: *Textbook of pediatric advanced life support,* 1990, American Heart Association and American Academy of Pediatrics, pp. 21-36.

[2]Aoki BY, McCloskey K: *Evaluation and stabilization and transport of the critically ill child,* St Louis, 1992, Mosby, pp. 1-16.

[3]Norwood SS: Respiratory emergencies. In Norwood SS, Zaritsky AL, eds.: *Guidelines to pediatric emergency care,* 1992, Emergency Medical Services for Children Project.

[4]Rowe PC, ed.: *The Harriet Lane handbook,* Chicago, 1987, Year Book, pp. 302-303.

Bag-Valve-Mask Ventilation

➤ **PURPOSE**

To adequately ventilate an infant or child with a bag-valve-mask device.

➤ **SUPPLIES**

Appropriate size ventilation bag device
- pediatric bag (500 ml tidal volume)
- adult bag (1000 ml tidal volume)

Appropriate size mask (should cover but not extend beyond the chin and bridge of the nose)
Nasogastric (NG) tube
Oxygen (O_2) source
Suction source
Nonsterile gloves
Goggles

➤ **PROCEDURE**

1. Determine the need for assisted ventilation by assessing the child's respiratory effort.
   Provide assisted ventilation if the infant or child has minimal or absent respiratory effort.

2. Wash hands.

3. Put on gloves and goggles. Maintain universal precautions throughout the procedure.

Fig 3-2

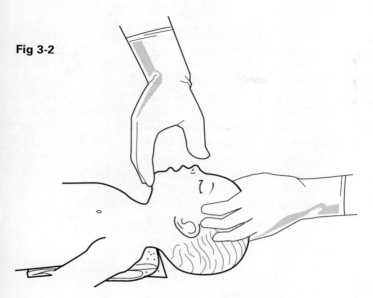

4. Open the child's airway using the head tilt–chin lift maneuver (Fig. 3-2). If a cervical spine injury is suspected, substitute the jaw thrust maneuver and perform spinal immobilization (Fig. 3-3).

Fig 3-3

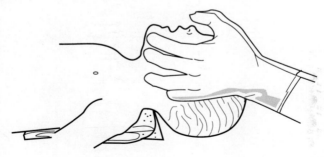

5. Assemble supplies. Select the appropriate ventilation bag
   device for the child (Fig. 3-4).

   *A self-inflating bag device is easier to use and is preferred
   over an anesthesia bag device.[1] Normal tidal volume for the
   intubated child is approximately 10 to 15 ml/kg. Neonatal
   size ventilation bags (250 ml) may not provide adequate
   tidal volume or prolonged inspiratory time for full-term
   newborns and infants, especially those with poorly compliant or atelectatic lungs. For this reason it is recommended
   that ventilation bags for full-term newborns, infants and
   children have a minimum tidal volume of 450 ml.[1,2] 250 ml
   ventilation bags are reserved for premature newborns.*

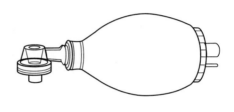

Fig 3-4

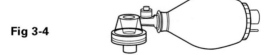

6. Attach the ventilation bag device to the O_2 source (Fig. 3-5). *An oxygen flow rate of at least 10 L/min is required to maintain an adequate volume in the ventilation bag.*[2]

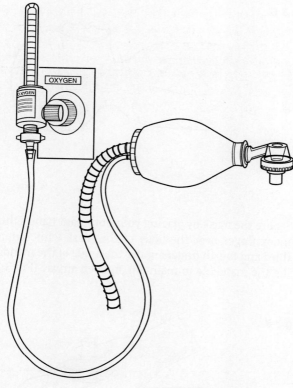

Fig 3-5

7. Place the appropriate size mask firmly on the face (Fig. 3-6).
   *The mask should have limited dead space, an inflatable rim,
   and should provide a tight seal without pressure on the eyes.*[2]

Fig 3-6

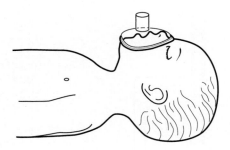

8. Secure the mask by placing your dominant hand's thumb and
   index finger over the body of the mask while cupping the
   third and fourth fingers under the angle of the mandible, lift-
   ing the mandible to maintain an open airway (Fig 3-7).

Fig 3-7

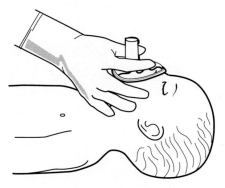

9. With the nondominant hand, attach the bag-valve ventilation device to the mask. Compress the ventilation bag slowly until chest rise is achieved (Fig. 3-8).

Fig 3-8

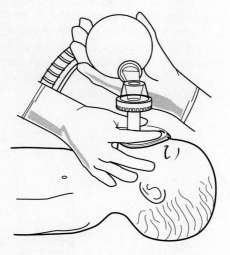

If an air leak is audible, this procedure may require two health care providers, one to maintain an open airway and mask seal and one to ventilate using the bag-valve device (Fig. 3-9). A bag with a pop-off valve requires two health care providers. A bag with a pop-off valve does not allow inspiratory pressures to exceed 40 cm H_2O pressure; however, higher inspiratory pressures are required during cardiopulmonary resuscitation and in patients with poor lung compliance.[2] Therefore one health care provider maintains an open airway and mask seal and the other depresses the pop-off valve and ventilates.

Fig 3-9

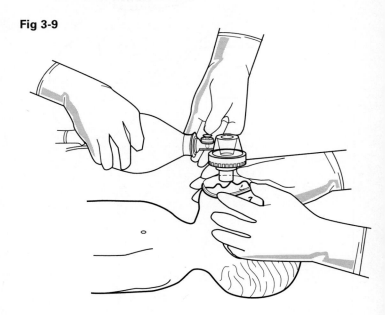

10. Release the bag and allow for complete expiration.

11. Continue to ventilate in this fashion until an artificial airway is placed or the child demonstrates adequate spontaneous ventilation.

    Initial rates of 20 to 30 breaths per minute for infants and 16 to 20 breaths per minute for children are adequate. Higher rates may be indicated if improvement is not observed.[2]

12. If bag-valve-mask ventilation is prolonged, place a nasogastric (NG) tube according to "Inserting Nasogastric (NG) and Orogastric (OG) Tubes" and attach the NG tube to intermittent suction.

    Pressure on the diaphragm from excess air in the stomach impedes ventilation.

13. Document need for and response to bag-valve-mask ventilation. Include the time frame of assisted ventilation.

References

[1]Todres IO: Pediatric airway control and ventilation, *Ann Emerg Med* 22 (pt. 2):440-444, 1993.

[2]Emergency Cardiac Care Committee and Subcommittees, American Heart Association: Guidelines for cardiopulmonary resuscitation and emergency cardiac care, VI: pediatric ACLS, *JAMA* 268:2262-2275, 1992.

Ventilation via an Endotracheal or Tracheostomy Tube

➤ **PURPOSE**

To adequately provide bag-valve ventilation via an endotracheal or tracheostomy tube.

➤ **SUPPLIES**

Appropriate size ventilation bag device

- pediatric bag (500 ml tidal volume)
- adult bag (1000 ml tidal volume)

Oxygen (O_2) source
Nonsterile gloves
Goggles

➤ **PROCEDURE**

1. Determine the need for bag-valve ventilation.
   Bag-valve ventilation via an endotracheal or tracheostomy tube is indicated in the following circumstances:

   - *the child is apneic or in respiratory failure*
   - *a mechanical ventilator is not available*
   - *the child's respiratory status is deteriorating on current ventilator settings*
   - *suctioning is required*

2. Wash hands.

3. Put on gloves and goggles. Maintain universal precautions throughout the procedure.

4. Select the appropriate ventilation bag device for the patient (Fig. 3-10).

A self-inflating bag device is easier to use and is preferred over an anesthesia bag device.[1] Normal tidal volume for the intubated child is approximately 10 to 15 ml/kg. Neonatal size (250 ml) ventilation bags may not provide adequate tidal volume or prolonged inspiratory time for full-term newborns and infants, especially those with poorly compliant or atelectatic lungs. For this reason it is recommended that ventilation bags for full-term newborns, infants, and children have a minimum tidal volume of 450 ml.[1,2] 250 ml ventilation bags are reserved for premature newborns.

Fig 3-10

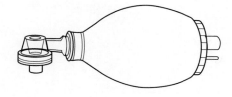

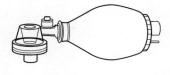

5. Attach the ventilation bag device to the O_2 source (Fig. 3-11). *An O_2 flow rate of at least 10 L/min is required to maintain adequate volume in the ventilation bag.*[2]

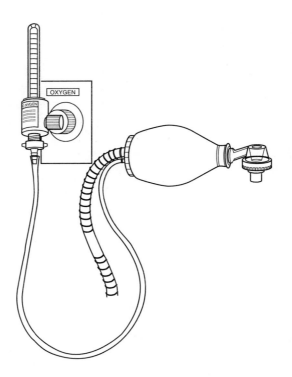

Fig 3-11

6. Attach the ventilation bag to the endotracheal or tracheostomy tube (Fig. 3-12).

Fig 3-12

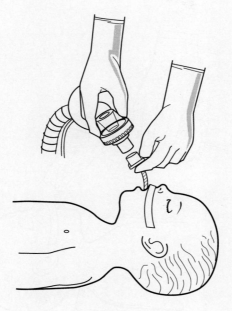

7. Slowly compress the ventilation bag until the chest rises (Fig. 3-13).

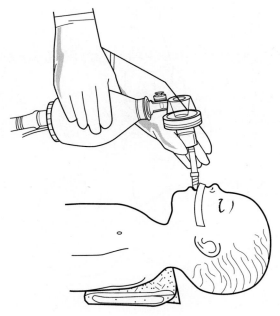

Fig 3-13

8. Release the bag and allow complete expiration.

9. Repeat Steps 7 and 8 at a rate appropriate for the child's age and respiratory status.
   Initial rates of 20 to 30 breaths per minute for infants and 16 to 20 breaths per minute for children are adequate. If the child has increased intracranial pressure or underlying pulmonary disease, higher rates may be needed.[2]

   If suctioning is required, refer to "Suctioning."

10. Discontinue bag-valve ventilation when a mechanical ventilator is available and the child's heart rate, oxygen saturation, skin color, and respiratory effort return to baseline (Fig. 3-14). (Some children with a tracheostomy tube may not require mechanical ventilator support.)

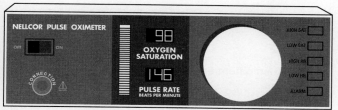

Fig 3-14

11. Ensure that the tape or ties securing the endotracheal or tracheostomy tube are adequate.

12. Document the need for and response to bag-valve ventilation.

References

[1]Todres IO: Pediatric airway control and ventilation, *Ann Emerg Med* 22(pt. 2):440-444, February 1993.

[2]Emergency Cardiac Care Committee and Subcommittees, American Heart Association: Guidelines for cardiopulmonary resuscitation and emergency cardiac care, VI: pediatric ACLS, *JAMA* 268:2262-2275, 1992.

Suctioning

➤ **PURPOSE**

To maintain patent artificial and natural airways by clearing secretions.

➤ **SUPPLIES**

Goggles
Sterile gloves
Sterile suction catheter
Normal saline (NS) for tracheal instillation
Suction source with gauge
Secretion trap with attached tubing
Appropriate size ventilation bag device

- pediatric bag (500 ml tidal volume)
- adult bag (1000 ml tidal volume)

Water soluble lubricant (nasotracheal suctioning)
Stethescope

➤ **GENERAL PROCEDURE**

1. Explain to the child and family the need for suctioning to maintain a patent airway. Be honest in explaining that it will be uncomfortable but will not take very long. Reassure the child throughout the procedure.

➤ **PROCEDURE—Endotracheal Tube (ETT)**

2. Determine the need for suctioning:

   • secretions are visible in the tube
   • airway pressures are increased
   • breath sounds are coarse

3. Assemble supplies.
   Catheter size varies according to the diameter of the artificial airway. Table 3-3 suggests the appropriate size for suction catheters.

Table 3-3 Suggested Suction Catheter Sizes	
ETT Size	**Recommended Suction Catheter Size**
2.5 mm	6.0 french
3.0 mm	6.0 french
3.5 mm	8.0 french
4.0 mm	8.0 french
4.5 mm	8.0 french
5.0 mm	10 french
5.5 mm	10 french

Modified from Runton N: Suctioning artificial airways in children: appropriate technique, *Pediatr Nurs* 18(2):117, 1992.

4. Procure assistance.
   The pediatric ETT is uncuffed and easily dislodged. Use two people for this procedure.

5. Wash hands.

6. Put on goggles. Maintain universal precautions throughout the procedure.

7. Connect secretion trap with attached tubing to the suction source. Adjust suction gauge to 80 mm Hg (Fig. 3-15).
Various levels of negative pressure are suggested. In general, negative pressures of 60 to 100 mm Hg are sufficient.[1] Higher pressures are associated with mucosal damage, atelectasis, and a decrease in lung compliance.[2,3]

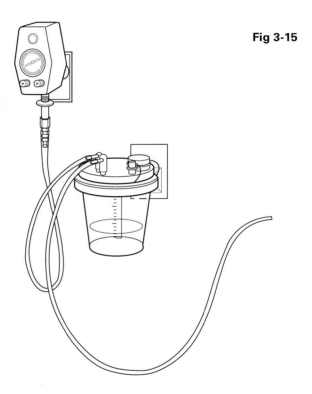

Fig 3-15

8. Connect the ventilation bag device to an O_2 source. Adjust the level of O_2 to 100% (Fig. 3-16).

Several recommendations have been made on the level of O_2 that is appropriate for preoxygenation. Children may be pre-oxygenated with 100% O_2[1] but this may have adverse effects on premature infants. Therefore 10% to 20% higher O_2 than baseline requirements is recommended for premature infants.[2,4,5]

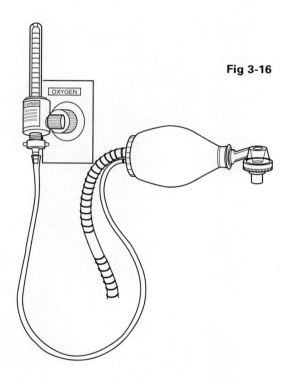

Fig 3-16

9. Open suction kit and put on sterile gloves. Maintain sterile technique. Grasp suction catheter with dominant hand, being careful not to contaminate the catheter. Attach the catheter to the suction tubing (Fig. 3-17).

   The dominant hand remains sterile throughout the procedure; the nondominant hand does not.

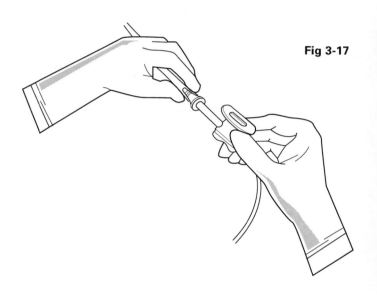

Fig 3-17

10. Note the child's heart rate, O_2 saturations (if available), and color.

11. Remove the ventilator tubing or ventilation bag device from the ETT (Fig. 3-18).

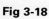

Fig 3-18

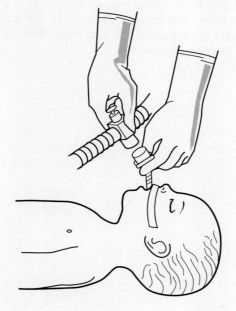

12. Instill NS (3 to 5 drops for infants, 0.5 ml for children, or 1.0 to 2.0 ml for adolescents)[1] into the ETT (Fig. 3-19).

Controversy exists regarding the use of NS as an irrigant before suctioning. NS has been associated with decreases in PaO_2 and its effectiveness in thinning secretions has been questioned.[1,5] However, considering the small diameter of pediatric ETTs, saline may be beneficial to prevent mucus from lining the internal diameter of the artificial airway.[1] Do NOT use intravenous NS, as it contains preservatives that will burn lung tissue.[1]

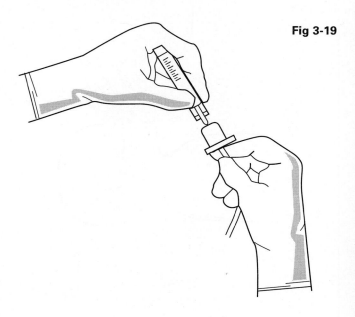

Fig 3-19

13. Attach the ventilation bag device and hyperventilate the patient with 5 to 10 manual breaths (Fig. 3-20). Watch for chest rise when bagging, being careful not to give too much volume.

    The concepts of hyperinflation and preoxygenation to minimize the effect of suction-induced atelectasis and hypoxemia have not been adequately evaluated in the pediatric population. It is recommended that the infant or child be given 5 to 10 breaths over 5 to 10 seconds before suctioning.[2,5]

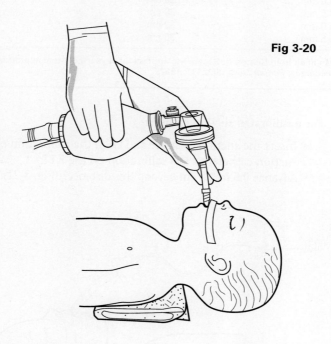

Fig 3-20

14. Remove the ventilation bag device.

15. Insert the suction catheter to the appropriate depth as outlined in Table 3-4.

Table 3-4 Length of Catheter to be Inserted during Suctioning	
ETT Size	**Length**
2.5 mm	20 cm
3.0 mm	23 cm
3.5 mm	25 cm
4.0 mm	28 cm
4.5 mm	30 cm
5.0 mm	32 cm
5.5 mm	35 cm

Modified from Runton N: Suctioning artificial airways in children: appropriate technique, *Pediatr Nurs* 18(2):117, 1992.

For a calibrated suction catheter:

• Insert the suction catheter and align the calibration of the suction catheter to the calibration on the ETT.
• Advance 0.5 to 1.0 cm beyond this distance[1] (Fig. 3-21).

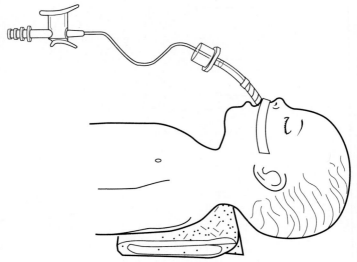

Fig 3-21

For a noncalibrated suction catheter:

- Measure the total length of a same sized ETT with a tape measure.
- Mark this spot on the tape measure.
- Attach the tape measure to the bed railing (Fig. 3-22).
- Using the tape measure as a reference, insert the suction catheter to the appropriate depth.

Fig 3-22

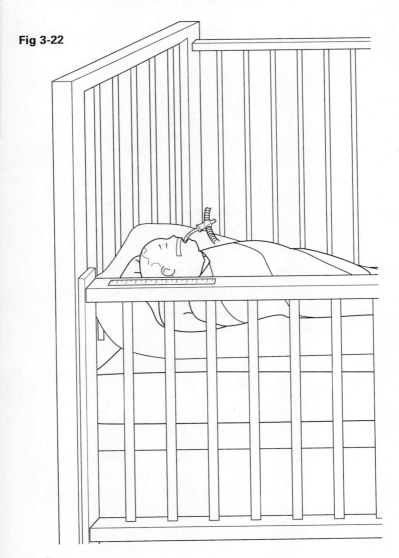

16. Apply suction and withdraw the catheter using a gentle rotating motion. Never suction for longer than 5 to 10 seconds.[1,5]

17. Attach ventilation bag device and manually ventilate for 30 seconds at a rate of 40 to 60/minute (Fig. 3-23).
    At least 30 seconds should be allotted between suction attempts to ensure reoxygenation and reperfusion.[1]

Fig 3-23

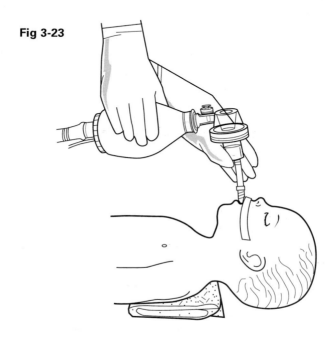

18. Repeat Steps 11 to 16, hyperventilating between each pass and monitoring the child's heart rate and color. (If available, monitor oxygen saturations by pulse oximeter during this procedure.)
The amount and character of secretions and the patient's tolerance of the procedure determine the number of times the catheter is passed.

19. Reattach the ventilator circuit to the ETT.

20. Discard the catheter and gloves.

21. Reevaluate heart rate, color, O_2 saturation, and breath sounds (Fig. 3-24).

22. Document character of secretions and child's response to suctioning.

23. Give the child positive feedback.

Fig 3-24

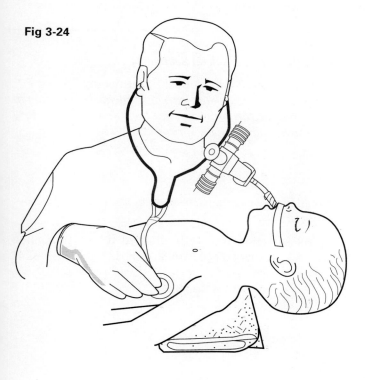

➤ *PROCEDURE—Tracheostomy Tube*

2. Follow the same procedure as ETT suctioning, taking care to introduce the catheter only 0.5 to 1.0 cm beyond the tip of the tracheostomy tube. Depths for tracheostomy tube suctioning are outlined in Table 3-5.

Table 3-5 Suggested Depth of Tracheostomy Tube Suctioning	
Shiley Size (Pediatric)	**Length of Catheter to be Inserted during Suctioning**
2.5 mm	6.0 cm
3.0 mm	6.0 cm
3.5 mm	6.0 cm
4.0 mm	6.0 cm
4.5 mm	6.5 cm
5.0 mm	6.5 cm
5.5 mm	7.0 cm

Modified from Runton N: Suctioning artificial airways in children: appropriate technique, *Pediatr Nurs* 18(2):117, 1992.

➤ *PROCEDURE—Nasotracheal Suctioning*

2. Determine the need for nasotracheal suctioning.
   Laryngospasm is associated with nasotracheal suctioning in infants. Reserve this procedure for the infant in respiratory distress with audible upper airway congestion.

3. Assemble supplies.

4. Wash hands.

5. Put on goggles. Maintain universal precautions throughout the procedure.

6. Connect secretion trap with attached tubing to suction source. Adjust suction gauge to 80 mm Hg.

7. Estimate depth to suction by holding the catheter beside the child's face, measuring from the tip of the nose to the ear (Fig. 3-25).

Fig 3-25

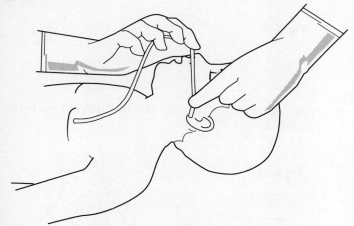

8. Apply water-soluble lubricant to the tip of the suction catheter (Fig. 3-26).

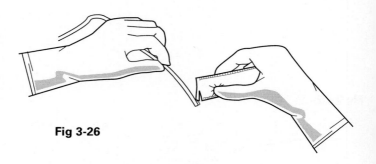

Fig 3-26

9. Gently introduce the catheter into the nasopharynx without applying suction (Fig. 3-27).

Fig 3-27

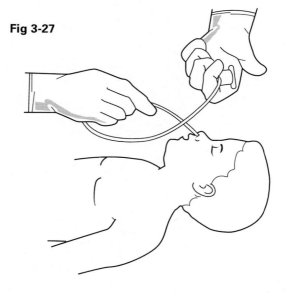

10. Apply suction to the catheter and withdraw.

11. Repeat Steps 9 and 10 until secretions are clear or minimal.

12. Discard gloves and catheter.

13. Document character of secretions and child's response to suctioning.

14. Give the child positive feedback.

References

[1]Runton N: Suctioning artificial airways in children: appropriate technique, *Pediatr Nurs* 18(2):115-118, 1992.

[2]Hodge D: Endotracheal suctioning and the infant: a nursing care protocol to decrease complications, *Neonatal Netw* 9(5):7-15, 1991.

[3]Wood RE: *Suctioning the pediatric artificial airway,* Chapel Hill, N.C., January 1990, University of North Carolina Hospitals.

[4]Shorten DR: Effects of tracheal suctioning on neonates: a review of the literature, *Intensive Care Nurs* 5(4):167-170, 1989.

[5]Turner BS: Maintaining the artificial airway: current concepts, *Pediatr Nurs* 16(5):487-493, 1990.

Securing an Endotracheal Tube (ETT)

➤ **PURPOSE**

To adequately secure the ETT and prevent the following complications:
- unplanned extubation with acute hypoxia and bradycardia
- right mainstem bronchus intubation
- esophageal intubation
- laryngotracheal damage

➤ **SUPPLIES**

Nonsterile gloves
1/2″ adhesive tape*
Benzoin
Alcohol swabs
Nonsterile gauze

➤ **PROCEDURE**

1. Assemble supplies.

2. Procure assistance. Taping a pediatric ETT always requires two health care providers, one to stabilize the child's head and ETT and the other to apply the tape.

3. Wash hands.

4. Put on gloves. Maintain universal precautions throughout the procedure.

---

*Several different types of tape have been recommended for use in securing an ETT: adhesive silk,[4,5] elastic tape,[4,6] waterproof tape,[6] and pink tape (water resistant and nonstretchable).[4] Maintenance of adhesive properties when exposed to saliva is the major criterion when selecting tape for ETT stabilization.

5. Tear tape in an "H-frame" (Fig. 3-28), leaving 1 cm for a bridge to ensure that the tape will not tear in half. The tape should reach from mid-cheek to mid-cheek but not cover the ears. *While several techniques have been developed for securing ETTs (e.g., Logan Bow and adhesive tape,[1] sutures through the ETT and tape,[1] modified umbilical clamp and safety pin,[2] and headstrap devices[3]), plain tape is the most accessible in an emergent intubation and, if applied correctly, suffices to secure the ETT.*

Fig 3-28

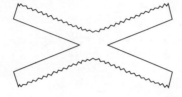

6. Tear a second piece of tape in a "Y-frame" (Fig. 3-29). Measure length as in Step 5.

Fig 3-29

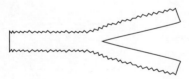

7. Explain to the child that you will be "taping this plastic tube." Explain that someone will place his or her hands on the child's forehead and chin to help hold them still.

8. Note the distance marker of the ETT at the lip level. Have a second health care provider hold the child's head and ETT by placing one hand on the forehead to prevent side-to-side movement, and cupping the palm of the other hand under the chin while securing the tube with the fingers (Fig. 3-30). *Consult with physician about sedation if the child is awake and moving. Movement of the child's head before the ETT is secured could dislodge it from the trachea.*

The position of oral tubes at the lip may be rapidly estimated through formulas such as:

- *3 × tube diameter*
- *age in years divided by 2 + 12*
- *weight in kg divided by 5 + 12[4]*

Fig 3-30

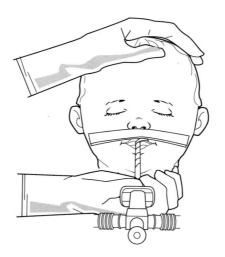

9. Assess breath sounds. If this is a newly placed tube, proceed to Step 11.

10. Loosen the tape by swabbing with alcohol. Remove the tape.

11. Clean and dry the area around the mouth with gauze pads (Fig. 3-31).

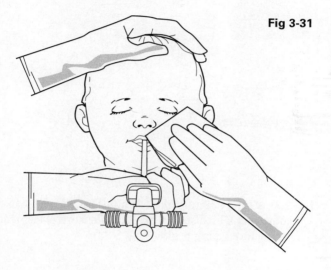

Fig 3-31

12. Apply benzoin to the area above upper lip and extending 1 to 2 cm laterally from the mouth. Allow to dry (Fig. 3-32).

Fig 3-32

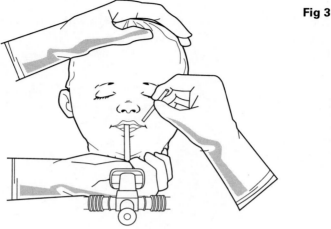

13. Assess for bilateral breath sounds, equal chest excursion, color, and ETT distance marker to ensure placement is correct before taping begins (Fig. 3-33).

Fig 3-33

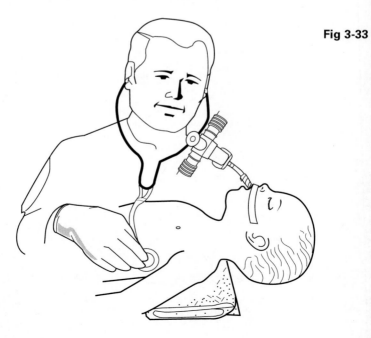

14. Place the upper portion of the H-frame on the upper lip area, and extend from cheek to cheek (Fig. 3-34).

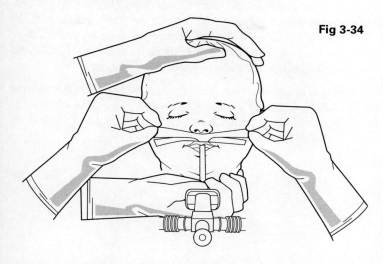

Fig 3-34

15. Check distance marker to ensure ETT is still in correct position.

16. Spiral one of the loose H-frame ends up the ETT, allowing 2 to 3 loops to be in direct contact with the ETT. Fold a small tab at the end of the tape to facilitate removal.

17. Spiral the second loose piece of tape on top of the first, again covering as much of the distance of the ETT as possible (Fig. 3-35). Fold a small tab at the end of the tape to facilitate removal.

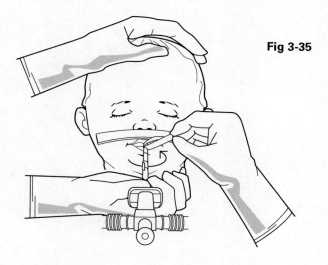

Fig 3-35

18. Place the Y-frame across the upper lip area extending cheek to cheek, leaving the bottom end free. Ensure that the fork in the tape is positioned immediately above the ETT (Fig. 3-36). *An alternative taping technique includes using two Y-frames.[4,5,7] This is done by securing a base on each side of the face and taping one tail clockwise around the ETT and the opposite tail counterclockwise around the ETT.*

Very little research has been done comparing the effectiveness of different taping techniques. One study found the H-frame to be significantly better then the Y-frame at preventing accidental extubations.[4]

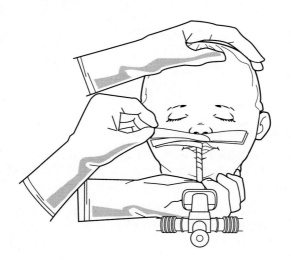

Fig 3-36

19. Spiral the free end of the Y-frame up the ETT. Fold a small tab at the end of the tape to facilitate removal.

20. Assess for bilateral breath sounds, equal chest excursion, and adequate color, indicating that the ETT is still placed correctly (Fig. 3-37).

21. Give the child positive feedback.

22. Document date and time of taping and correlation of the ETT's distance marker with the child's lip.

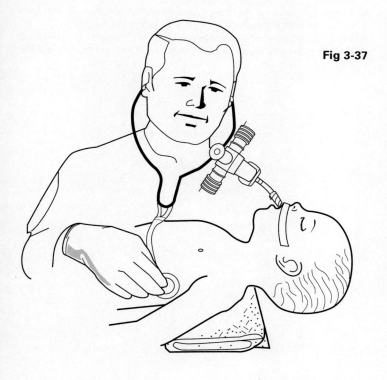

Fig 3-37

References

[1]Budd RA: The "Logan Bow" method for securing endotracheal tubes in neonates, *Crit Care Nurse* 2(3):27-28, 1982.

[2]Nieves J: Avoiding spontaneous extubation of nasotracheal or oral tracheal tubes, *Pediatr Nurs* 12(3):215-218, 1986.

[3]Tasota FJ et al: Evaluation of two methods to stabilize oral endotracheal tubes, *Heart Lung* 19:140-146, 1987.

[4]Brown MS: Prevention of accidental extubation in newborns, *Am J Dis Child* 142:1240-1243, 1988.

[5]Hughes WT, Buescher ES: *Pediatric procedures,* ed 2, Philadelphia, 1981, WB Saunders.

[6]Robson LK, Tompkins J: Maintaining placement and skin integrity with endotracheal tubes in a pediatric ICU, *Crit Care Nurse* 4(3):29-32, 1984.

[7]Christoph RA: Pulmonary and cardiac resuscitation procedures. In Lohr JA, ed.: *Pediatric outpatient procedures,* Philadelphia, 1991, JB Lippincott, pp. 305-339.

Medication Delivery via an Endotracheal Tube (ETT)

➤ **PURPOSE**

To deliver medications via an ETT when there is no vascular access.

➤ **SUPPLIES**

Appropriate size ventilation bag device

- pediatric bag (500 ml tidal volume)
- adult bag (1000 ml tidal volume)

Appropriate dose of correct medication
Oxygen (O_2) source
Two 3 ml syringes
Normal saline (NS) or sterile water
5 F feeding tube
Adhesive tape
Sterile gloves
Goggles
Extra ETT of the same size

➤ **PROCEDURE**

1. Assemble supplies. Select the appropriate ventilation bag device (see "Bag-Valve-Mask Ventilation").

2. Procure assistance.

3. Wash hands.

4. Put on gloves and goggles. Maintain universal precautions throughout the procedure.

5. Draw correct dose of appropriate medication into a 3 ml syringe.

The following medications may be administered via the artificial airway:

- *Lidocaine (1 mg/kg)*
- *Atropine (0.02 mg/kg) [minimum dose = 0.1 mg, maximum dose = 0.5 mg]*
- *Naloxone (0.01 mg/kg)*
- *Epinephrine (0.1 mg/kg using 1:1000 concentration)*

Optimal drug doses for endotracheal administration remain unknown, as absorption is erratic. Studies show that peak epinephrine levels after endotracheal administration are only one tenth of the peak levels following intravenous administration.[1,2] As a result, the American Heart Association now recommends that the initial dose of epinephrine endotracheally be 0.1 mg/kg (100 mcg/kg).[3] This is ten times the IV dose. Doses of other resuscitation drugs should also be increased when given endotracheally.[3]

6. Dilute the medication to a total volume of 2 ml with normal saline.
   Data conflict regarding the optimal amount of diluent. If the drug will be administered through a catheter placed in the ETT, the drug should be administered in a total volume of at least 2 ml.[4]

   NS is an appropriate diluent for epinephrine, atropine, and naloxone. Lidocaine is better absorbed if diluted with sterile water.[5]

7. Determine the depth of insertion for the feeding tube.

- Open the feeding tube package maintaining sterile technique.
- Put on sterile gloves.
- Insert the feeding tube into the extra ETT, aligning the tips.
- Place a piece of tape on the feeding tube where it matches the ETT adapter (Fig. 3-38).

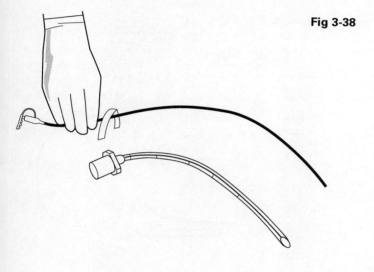

Fig 3-38

8. Have another health care provider attach the ventilation ba
device to the artificial airway and administer 2 to 3 breath
before medication delivery (Fig. 3-39). He or she then de
taches the ventilation bag device.

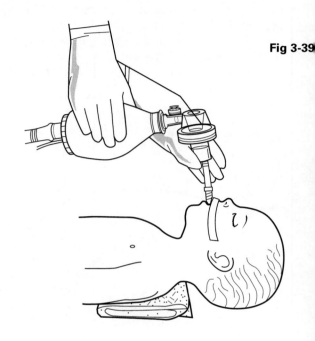

Fig 3-39

9. Insert the feeding tube through the artificial airway until the tape marking is at the level of the ETT adapter.

10. Instill the medication into the feeding tube (Fig. 3-40), then flush the feeding tube with 2 ml of air. This may increase drug delivery from the tube to the lungs.[6]
Although the best method for endotracheal drug delivery is not certain, delivery into the distal airways improves absorption.[7,8] If a catheter is not available to pass down the ETT, the drug may be administered directly into the ETT and followed with 2 to 5 ml of NS flush.[4]

Fig 3-40

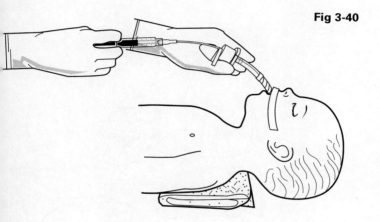

11. Withdraw the feeding tube and maintain sterile technique.

12. Have the other health care provider reattach the ventilation bag device and administer 5 breaths (Fig. 3-41).

13. Repeat Steps 9 to 12 for each medication to be administered.

14. Discard the feeding tube after all medications have been given via the ETT.

15. Document your name, the time, medicine, dose, and route of administration.

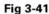

Fig 3-41

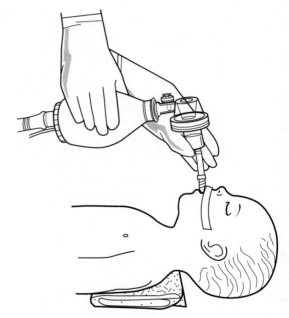

References

[1] Roberts JR et al: Blood levels following intravenous and endotracheal epinephrine administration, *JACEP* 8:53-56, 1979.

[2] Ralston S et al: Endotracheal versus intravenous epinephrine during electromechanical dissociation with CPR in dogs, *Ann Emerg Med* 14:1044-1048, 1985.

Emergency Cardiac Care Committee and Subcommittees, American Heart Association: Guidelines for cardiopulmonary resuscitation and emergency cardiac care, VI: pediatric ALS, *JAMA* 268:2262-2275, 1992.

[4] Zaritsky A: Pediatric resuscitation pharmacology, *Ann Emerg Md* 22(2) part 2:445-455, 1993.

[5] H?hnel J et al. Plasma lidocaine levels and PaO$_2$ with endobronchial administration: dilution with normal saline or distilled water? *Ann Emerg Med* 19:1314-1317, 1990.

[6] Johnston C: Endotracheal drug delivery, *Pediatric Emerg Care* 8(2):94-97, 1992.

[7] Ralston SH, Voorhees WD, Babbs CF: Intrapulmonary epinephrine during prolonged cardiopulmonary resuscitation: improved regional blood flow and resuscitation in dogs, *Ann Emerg Med* 13:79-86, 1984.

[8] Mazkereth R et al: Epinephrine blood concentrations after peripheral bronchial versus endotracheal administration of epinephrine in dogs, *Crit Care Med* 20(11), 1992.

Reinserting a Tracheostomy Tube

➤ **PURPOSE**

To quickly and safely apply appropriate techniques for re-inserting an obstructed or dislodged pediatric tracheostomy tube.

➤ **SUPPLIES**

Appropriate size pediatric tracheostomy tube
Pediatric tracheostomy tube one size smaller
Water-soluble lubricant or normal saline
Twill tape
Scissors
Appropriate size suction catheter

➤ **PROCEDURE**

1. Determine the need for reinserting the tracheostomy tube.
   Acute dislodgment of the tracheostomy tube may produce severe respiratory distress. It will be obvious if the tube has come completely out; however, the tube may remain in the neck but not in the trachea, making assessment difficult.

   Changing the tracheostomy tube is also necessary if the tube becomes obstructed with thick secretions or blood.

2. Assemble supplies.
   Tracheostomy tubes are made of either metal or plastic. Plastic pediatric tracheostomy tubes are frequently used and vary in length and internal diameter.[1] Table 3-6 lists pediatric tracheostomy tube sizes.

	Size	Internal Size (mm)	Outer Diameter (mm)	Length (mm)
Neonatal	00	3.1	4.5	30
	0	3.4	5.0	32
	1	3.7	5.5	34
Pediatric	00	3.1	4.5	39
	0	3.4	5.0	40
	1	3.7	5.5	41
	2	4.1	6.0	42
	3	4.8	7.0	44
	4	5.5	8.0	46

Table 3-6   Neonatal and Pediatric Tracheostomy Tube Sizes

3. Procure assistance.
   Changing the tracheostomy tube in an infant or child requires two people.[2,3,4]

4. Explain the procedure to the child and family if appropriate. Acute dislodgment or obstruction of the tracheostomy tube usually is a respiratory emergency, in which case explanations are brief at best.

5. Wash hands.

6. Put on gloves. Maintain universal precautions throughout the procedure.

7. Position the infant in a supine position with a towel roll under his or her neck and shoulders (Fig. 3-42). Instruct the other health care provider to hold the infant's neck, shoulders, and arms still.

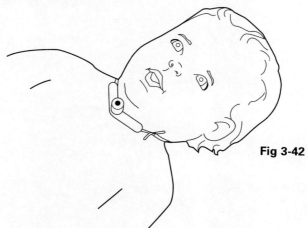

Fig 3-42

8. Insert the obturator into the new tube.

9. Lubricate the new tube with a small amount of sterile saline or a water-soluble lubricant. Handle the new tube by the wings or barrel, with your finger over the obturator to keep it in place (Fig. 3-43).

Fig 3-43

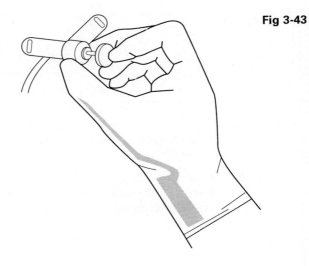

10. Remove the original tube.

    If the original tracheostomy tube is completely out of the neck, have the other health care provider cut the twill tape and remove the tube.

    If the original tracheostomy tube is still in the neck, have the other health care provider cut the twill tape and hold the tube in place until you are ready with the new tube.

11. Insert the new tube gently and quickly, with the curve of the tube following the downward curve of the trachea (Fig. 3-44). Immediately remove the obturator while holding the outer cannula in place.

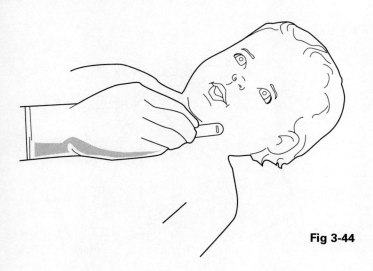

Fig 3-44

12. If unable to recannulate the trachea, try one of the following:

- Relubricate the tube, reposition the head, and try again using gentle pressure.[2,4]
- Attempt cannulation in the same manner with a tracheostomy tube one size smaller.[4]
- Insert a sterile suction catheter into the stoma and cut it off about 6 inches above the stoma. Do not let go of the catheter! Thread the new tube over the catheter and into the stoma (Fig. 3-45). Remove the catheter. If the tube still will not thread, leave the catheter in place and contact the child's physician.[2,4]

Fig 3-45

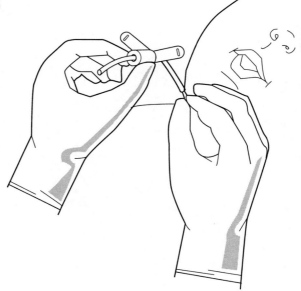

13. Observe for correct placement of the tube by assessing the infant's:
    • chest movement
    • color
    • vital signs
    • breath sounds.

14. Oxygenate and/or suction if necessary. Hold the tube in place until you can secure it with twill tape.

15. Thread twill tape through one wing of the tube and double it over.

16. Wrap the ties around the neck and thread one end of the twill tape through the other wing of the tube.

17. Tie the ends on the side of the neck with a square knot. Allow room for one finger to fit under the twill tape (Fig. 3-46).

18. Give the child positive feedback.

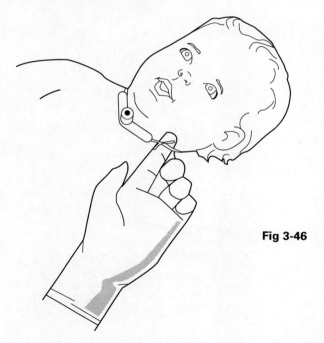

Fig 3-46

References

[1]Norwood SS: Respiratory emergencies. In Norwood SS, Zaritsky AL, eds.: *Guidelines for pediatric emergency care,* 1993, Emergency Medical Services for Children Project.

[2]Hazinski MF: Pediatric home tracheostomy care: a parent's guide, *Pedtr Nurs* 12(1):41-8, 69, 1986.

[3]Carabott J et al: Teaching families tracheostomy care, *Can Nurse* 87(3):21-22, 1991.

[4]Roemer NR: The tracheostomized child, *Home Health Nurse* 10(4):28-32, 1992.

Stabilization Procedures

Pediatric Spinal Immobilization

➤ **PURPOSE**

To apply appropriate spinal immobilization techniques to the pediatric patient.

➤ **SUPPLIES**

Nonsterile gloves
Long backboard with straps
Commercially available pediatric immobilizer
Towel rolls
Semi-rigid cervical collar
1¹/₂" to 2" adhesive tape

➤ **PROCEDURE**

1. Determine the need for spinal immobilization. Spinal immobilization is indicated in the infant or child who:

   • is unconscious
   • has sustained injuries to either the head or upper body
   • complains of pain in the head, neck, or back
   • has a neurological deficit resulting from an injury
   • was involved in an acceleration/deceleration accident
   • was the victim of a fall
   • was the victim of a diving accident
   • was the victim of child abuse

2. Put on gloves. Maintain universal precautions throughout the procedure.

3. Procure assistance.

4. Stand behind the child and stabilize the head in a neutral in-line position.

• Place your hands on both sides of the child's head, with your fingers on the occiput extending up the angle of the jaw (Fig. 4-1).

Traction is not recommended as it may cause damage to the immature spine, particularly if there is already damage to the area.[1,2,3]

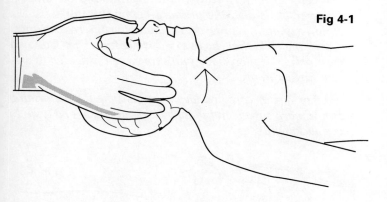

Fig 4-1

• If the child is moving, grasp him or her by the shoulders, immobilizing the head between your forearms (Fig. 4-2).

Fig 4-2

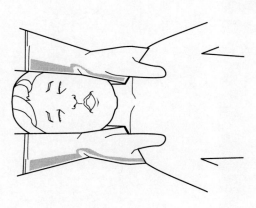

3. Maintain the airway by using the jaw-thrust maneuver (Fig. 4-3).

Do not use the head tilt–chin lift maneuver on any pediatric trauma victim.[3]

One health care provider is responsible for maintaining in-line cervical immobilization and maintaining the airway. This person is also the primary communicator with the child, explaining procedures and offering reassurance. Assure the child that the injury was not his or her fault and that immobilization is not punishment but is needed to prevent further injury.

Another health care provider is responsible for performing the primary survey and immobilizing the body and head to the backboard.

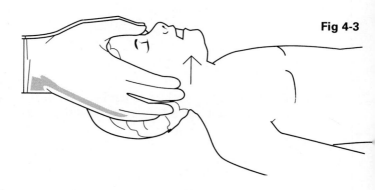

Fig 4-3

4. Perform a brief neurological exam on the child.

5. Apply a cervical collar while maintaining manual immobilization (Fig. 4-4).

   A Philadelphia collar may be used for children older than four if the child's chin fits into the chin groove in neutral position. Many of these collars are too large for children and will cause the neck to flex if the chin does not fit into the groove. The sides of the collar should not cover the ears.[1]

   If the right size collar is not available, make a soft collar with a rolled towel or sheet.

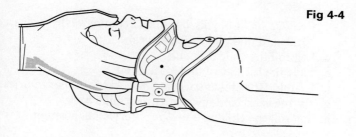

Fig 4-4

6. Place the child on the backboard.* While maintaining manual immobilization:

   a. Place the backboard next to the child.
   b. For an infant, place a small towel roll on the backboard at the level of the shoulders (Fig. 4-5).

   Infants have large occiputs that may cause the neck to flex when laid flat, producing undesirable cervical flexion.[4]

---

* Refer to the operator's manual if using a commercially available pediatric immobilizer. Although the principles remain the same, some steps may differ.

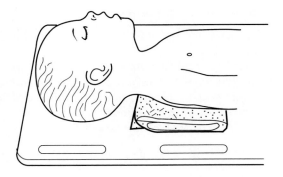

Fig 4-5

c. Remove foam blocks if using a commercially prepared backboard immobilization device.
d. Log roll the child as a unit.
e. Slide the backboard under the child.
f. Examine the child's back and buttocks for other injuries.
g. Tilt the backboard up to meet the child's back.
h. Log roll the child as a unit to a horizontal position.

7. Secure the child's body to the backboard before securing head.[5] Use at least three straps to immobilize the body in line with the head and neck (Fig. 4-6).
The straps may be applied straight across or the upper two may be crisscrossed over the torso.[1,2] If using an adult board, place towel or blanket rolls along the body to prevent lateral movement.[5]

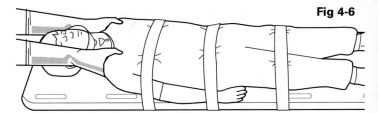

Fig 4-6

8. Place rolled towels or foam pads on either side of the child's head so they are resting against the side of the face and head (Fig. 4-7).
   Sandbags and IV bags on either side of the head are not recommended; the weight of the bags may cause movement of the head or neck if the board is tilted.[6]

Fig 4-7

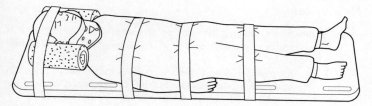

9. Tape with 1½" to 2" inch tape across the forehead, securing the towels or foam pads to the head and attaching each end of the tape to the board (Fig. 4-7).
   Do not put a gauze pad on the child's forehead to prevent the tape from sticking to the forehead. The purpose of this tape is to immobilize the child's head and neck.

   Do not place tape across the chin; this may cause the airway to become occluded. If extra support is needed, place tape across the bridge between the upper lip and the nose, attaching each end of the tape to the board.

10. Discontinue manual in-line positioning when the child's head and body are immobilized securely.

11. Maintain a patent airway.
    When an infant or child lies on his or her back, the tongue may relax and occlude the airway.

12. Repeat a brief neurological exam.
    Note any changes in the child's neurological status that may be the result of immobilization.

13. Maintain the child's body temperature; encircle the child with blankets, covering the top of the head, and, if possible, turn up the heat in the vehicle or emergency room.
Infants and children are especially prone to hypothermia, which will cause their condition to deteriorate.

14. Give the child positive feedback.

References

[1]Lang S: Procedures involving the neurological system. In Bernardo L, Bove M, eds.: *Pediatric emergency nursing procedures,* Boston, 1993, Jones & Bartlett, pp. 143-161.

[2]Runge JW: Orthopedic problems in pediatric trauma. In Hamilton JP, Jacobs A, Morton D, eds.: *Pediatric trauma management for emergency medical services,* Charlotte, NC, 1989, Hemby Pediatric Trauma Institute, pp. 53-59.

[3]Emergency Cardiac Care Committee and Subcommittees, American Heart Association: Guidelines for cardiopulmonary resuscitation and emergency cardiac care, V: pediatric BLS, *JAMA* 285:2251-2261, 1992.

[4]Hersenberg JE et al: Emergency transport and positioning of younger children who have an injury of the cervical spine, *J Bone Joint Surg Am* 71-A(1):15-22, 1989.

[5]Immobilization techniques for neck and spine trauma. In *Advanced trauma life support student manual,* Chicago, 1993, American College of Surgeons, pp. 211-218.

[6]Norwood SS: Pediatric trauma. In Norwood SS, Zaritsky AL, eds.: *Guidelines for pediatric emergency care,* 1992, Emergency Medical Services for Children Project.

Temperature Assessment

➤ **PURPOSE**

To determine the most appropriate temperature technique for the child's age and condition, then apply the correct technique.

➤ **SUPPLIES**

Thermometer: mercury, electronic, or tympanic
Nonsterile gloves
Water-soluble lubricant
Hospital-approved equipment cleaning solution

➤ **PROCEDURE**

1. Choose the appropriate method for the child's age and condition, as shown in the boxes on pp. 144-147.

2. When appropriate, explain to the child and/or family the need for an accurate temperature measurement.

3. Allow the child to maintain a position of comfort, possibly on parent's lap.

4. Wash hands.

5. Put on gloves. Maintain universal precautions throughout the procedure.

6. Take the child's temperature according to the guidelines in the boxes on pp. 144-147.

7. Intervene if core temperature is < 36° C (96.8° F) or > 38.5° C (101.4° F).

8. Give the child positive feedback.

9. Reassess every 30 minutes to 1 hour if abnormal.

Route **Recommended Use**	• Axillary
	• Neonates[1]
	• Uncooperative children who are not suspected of having a fever and who may view rectal temperatures as threatening[2]
Recommended Thermometer	• Mercury[2,3]–mercury thermometers can measure 34° to 42° C (94° to 107° F)
Notes	• Electronic thermometers are not accurate for determining fever using axillary route[2]
	• The axillary route is preferred in neonates because it:
	a. avoids the risk of bowel perforation
	b. reflects heat or cold stress sooner as skin temperature drops before core temperature drops
	c. causes minimal stimulation to the neonate.[1]
Guidelines	1. Shake down thermometer until mercury is below 35.5° C (96° F).
	2. Hold thermometer in axilla skin fold for 3 minutes.[1,4]
	3. Clean thermometer with hospital-approved cleaning solution.
Relationship to Core Temperature	• 1° C less[5]

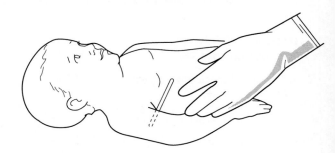

Route	• Oral
Recommended Use	• Children 5 years and older[3]
	• Cooperative children
	• Children with normal level of consciousness[3]
Recommended Thermometer	• Electronic[2,3]—electronic thermometers can measure as low as 34.5° C (94° F)
Notes	• Oral temperature accuracy is affected by increased respiratory rate and oral fluid intake.
	• Do not use mercury thermometers for preschoolers; they may bite the thermometer and swallow contents.[3]
	• Taking temperature orally provides for the child's dignity and privacy.[3]
Guidelines	1. Place probe cover over electronic thermometer probe.
	2. Hold probe under tongue until signal is heard (approximately 20 to 30 seconds).
	3. Discard probe cover.
	4. If mercury thermometer is used, hold it under tongue for 3 to 5 minutes.[6,7]
	5. Clean off either type with hospital-approved cleaning solution.
Relationship to Core Temperature	• 0.6° C less

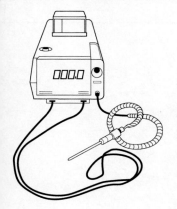
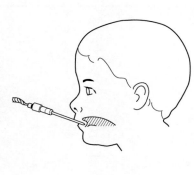

Route	• Rectal
Recommended Use	• Any infant or child with suspected fever[9] • Any infant or child with suspected hypothermia • Newborn admission[1,8]
Recommended Thermometer	• Electronic[2,3]—electronic thermometers can measure as low as 34.5° C (94° F)
Notes	• Rectal temperature measures the core temperature. • Hypothermia or hyperthermia require a core temperature. • Rectal temperatures are contraindicated for children with diarrhea.[7]
Guidelines	1. Place probe cover over electronic thermometer probe. 2. Lubricate the tip of the probe cover with water soluble jelly, e.g., KY jelly. 3. Place thermometer into rectum 2 cm for an infant or 4 cm for older child and hold until signal is heard. 4. Discard probe cover. 5. If mercury thermometer is used, hold in place for two minutes. 6. Clean thermometer with hospital-approved cleaning solution
Relationship to Core Temperature	• Equal

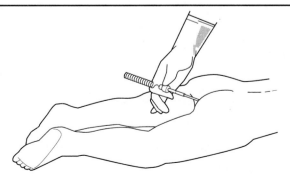

Route	• Tympanic
Recommended Use	• Children 3 years and older[9]
Recommended Thermometer	• Tympanic—measured ranges vary between manufacturers
Notes	• Tympanic route is not accurate in neonates.[6,9,10] • Tympanic temperature accuracy may be affected by ear wax.[6] • Tympanic route may be more acceptable to patients than rectal method.
Guidelines	1. Place probe cover over ear specula. 2. Pull outer ear back and insert instrument into one third of the external ear canal. 3. Hold in place until signal is heard (2 seconds). 4. Discard probe cover and clean with hospital-approved cleaning solution.
Relationship to Core Temperature	• If well controlled, should be equal

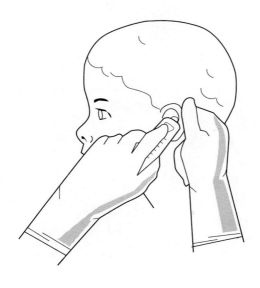

References

[1]Stephen SB: Neonatal axillary temperatures: increases in readings over time, *Neonatal Netw* 5(6):25-28, 1987.

[2]Ogren JM: The inaccuracy of axillary temperatures measured with an electronic thermometer, *Am J Dis Child* 144(1):109-111, 1990.

[3]Martyn KK: Comparison of axillary, rectal and skin-based temperature assessment in preschoolers, *Nurse Prac* 13(4):31-36, 1988.

[4]Hunter LP: Measurement of axillary temperatures in neonates, *West J Nurs Res* 13(3):324-335, 1991.

[5]Pilchak TM: Anesthesia and monitoring equipment for pediatrics, *CRNA* 3(2), 1992.

[6]Nobell JJ: Infrared ear thermometry, *Pediatr emerg care* 8(1):54-61, 1992.

[7]Skale N: *Manual of pediatric nursing procedures,* Philadelphia, 1992, Lippincott, pp. 28-34, 98-102.

[8]University of North Carolina Children's Hospital neonatal ICU thermoregulation guideline, Aug 1990.

[9]Davis K: The accuracy of tympanic temperature measurement in children, *Pediatr Nurs* 19(3):267-272, 1993.

[10]Chamberlain JM: Comparison of tympanic thermometer to rectal and oral thermometers in a pediatric emergency department, *Clin Pediatr* 30(4):24-29, 1991 (suppl).

Using Radiant Warmers

➤ **PURPOSE**

To use a radiant warmer safely to provide a warmed environment for newborns and infants.

➤ **SUPPLIES**

Radiant warmer or radiant warmer bed
Temperature probe and a reflective thermal probe cover
Linens
Manufacturer's instructions for use (each brand of warmer
  may have slightly different labels on control panel)

➤ **PROCEDURE**

1. Determine the need for a radiant warmer.
   *Radiant warmer beds (Fig. 4-8) are used for infants who are
   shorter than the bed's mattress, unable to roll over, and in
   need of stabilization or resuscitation procedures.[1] Radiant
   warmers (Fig. 4-9) should be used for any size pediatric
   patient requiring stabilization. Newborn and infants require
   a neutral thermal environment to minimize their oxygen
   consumption and caloric usage.*

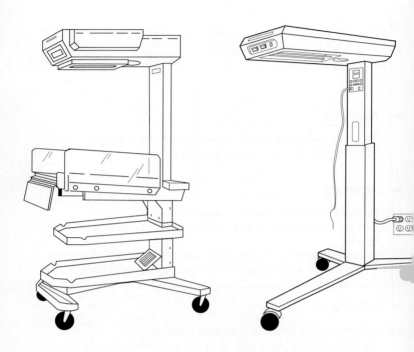

Fig 4-8   **Fig 4-9**

2. Explain to the family the need to use a radiant warmer to increase or maintain the infant's temperature.

3. Wash hands.

4. Plug warmer in and turn on.

5. Place the radiant warmer away from air conditioning flow currents.[2]
Radiant warmers lose the most heat by convection, *or cool air currents. Air movement also causes evaporative loss.*[3]

6. Prewarm the radiant warmer and linens.

   • Set heating control unit on "manual."
   • Increase output to 100% power (Fig. 4-10).

   Preheating the linens will decrease heat loss through conduction, *or loss of heat due to direct contact of infant's skin with cooler objects.*[4]

Fig 4-10

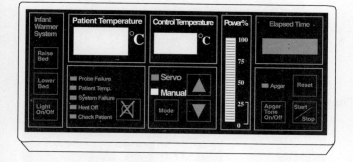

7. Change the heating control unit to "servo control" after the radiant warmer is preheated (Fig. 4-11).
Servo control adjusts the amount of heater output to maintain a constant skin temperature.

NEVER LEAVE AN INFANT UNDER A RADIANT WARMER ON MANUAL CONTROL. HYPERTHERMIA AND BURNS COULD OCCUR!

Fig 4-11

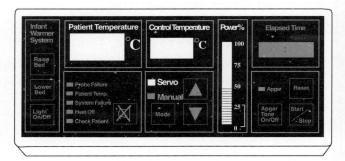

8. Set "control temperature" window at 37.0° C (98.6° F) (Fig. 4-12).

Fig 4-12

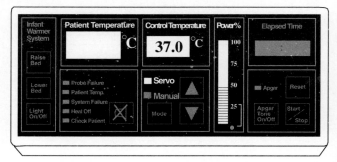

9. Place the undressed infant on the bed under the radiant heat. *Covered infants won't receive heat from a radiant warmer.*[4]

10. Plug the temperature probe into the warmer.

11. Place the flat metal side of the temperature probe against the infant's skin over the liver or in the axilla,[3] and cover probe end with a reflective thermal cover (Fig. 4-13).

Fig 4-13

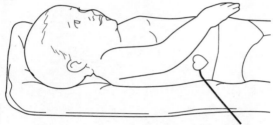

The probe will provide a continuous reading of the infant's skin temperature on the control panel (Fig. 4-14). The bed alarm will sound if the infant's skin probe temperature reading is more than 1° C different than the control temperature. If the probe comes off the infant's skin, the bed alarm will also sound.

Fig 4-14

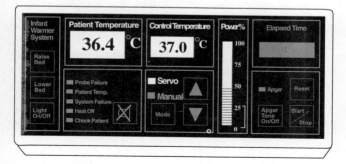

12. Immediately take infant's axillary temperature manually when he or she is put under warmer; repeat in 15 minutes (Fig. 4-15).

    If the second axillary temperature is too high or too low (see "Temperature Assessment"), adjust the "control temperature" in 0.5° C increments. Manually retake axillary temperature every 30 minutes to 1 hour until two successive normal temperatures are obtained (37° C or 98.6 ° F).

Fig 4-15

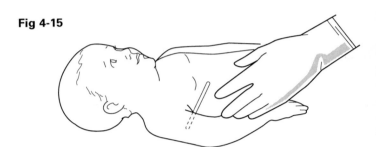

13. Record the "control temperature" reading and "patient temperature" reading hourly, as well as manual axillary temperature every 2 hours.

References

[1]Liebermon AB: *The preemie parent's handbook,* New Yor, 1984, Dutton, pp. 46-47.

[2]Whaley LF, Wong DL: *Nursing care of infants and children,* St Louis, 1979, Mosby, pp. 252-253, 338.

[3]Korones SB: *High-risk newborn infants,* St Louis, 1986, Mosby, pp. 90-93.

[4]Perez RH: *Protocols for perinatal nursing practice,* St Louis, 1981, Mosby, pp. 259-265.

Using an Isolette

➤ **PURPOSE**

To use an isolette safely to provide a warmed environment for infants.

➤ **SUPPLIES**

Isolette
Temperature probe and reflective thermal probe cover
Linens
Manufacturer's instructions for use (each brand of isolette may have slightly different labels on control panel)

➤ **PROCEDURE**

1. Determine the need for an isolette.
   Using an isolette for small babies provides the warmed environment that will minimize their oxygen consumption, caloric usage, and insensible water loss.[1] If the patient requires many procedures, resuscitation, or unobstructed observation, use a radiant warmer (see "Using Radiant Warmers").

2. Explain to the family the need to use an isolette to increase or maintain the infant's temperature.

3. Wash hands.

4. Plug isolette in and turn it on (Fig. 4-16).

Fig 4-16

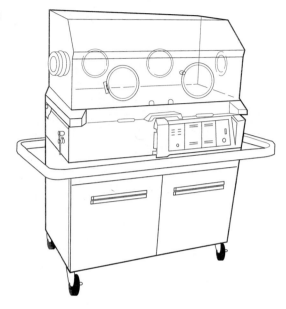

5. Place isolette away from windows and air conditioning units, which will cool the walls of the isolette.

Heat loss occurs through radiation, *or loss of heat to cooler solid objects in the environment that are not in direct contact with the infant.[2,3,4] A double-walled isolette further decreases the effects of the environment on the patient's temperature and is used with preterm or very small infants.[3]*

6. Prewarm the isolette and linens before placing infant inside. Set "air temperature" to 37° C (98.6° F) (Fig. 4-17).
Prewarming prevents heat loss through conduction, or loss of heat from direct contact of infant's skin to cooler objects.[4]

Fig 4-17

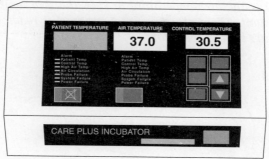

7. When the "control temperature" window and the "air temperature" window both read 37° C (98.6° F) (Fig. 4-18), place the undressed infant inside the isolette.
An isolette allows observation of the undressed infant, which is preferable to trying to observe an infant that is dressed and wrapped in blankets.[5]

Fig 4-18

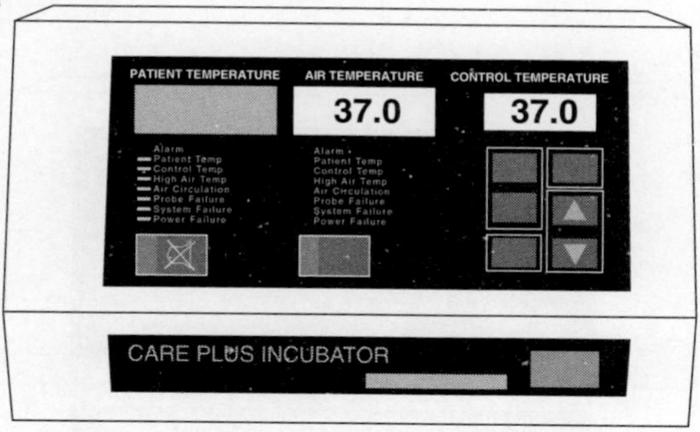

8. Plug the temperature probe into the isolette.

9. Place the flat metal side of the temperature probe against the infant's skin over the liver or in the axilla.[3] Cover probe end with a reflective thermal cover (Fig. 4-19).

   Use of a skin probe allows "patient control" thermoregulation (sometimes referred to as "servo control"), which adjusts the air temperature to keep the skin temperature constant. The probe provides a continuous reading of the infant's skin temperature.

Fig 4-19

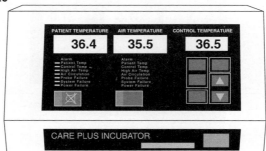

10. In the "patient control" mode, set the "control temperature" window to 36.5° C (97.7° F) (Fig. 4-20). The "control temperature" window now indicates the goal temperature for the infant's skin.

Fig 4-20

PATIENT TEMPERATURE   AIR TEMPERATURE   CONTROL TEMPERATURE
36.4   35.5   36.5

Alarm   Alarm
Patient Temp   Patient Temp
Control Temp   Control Temp
High Air Temp   High Air Temp
Air Circulation   Air Circulation
Probe Failure   Probe Failure
System Failure   System Failure
Power Failure   Power Failure

CARE PLUS INCUBATOR

11. Manually take the patient's axillary temperature (Fig. 4-21). If too high or too low (see "Temperature Assessment"), adjust "control temperature" by 0.2° C (0.1° F). Retake manual axillary temperature every 30 minutes to 1 hour until two successive normal temperatures are obtained (37.0° C or 98.6° F).

Fig 4-21

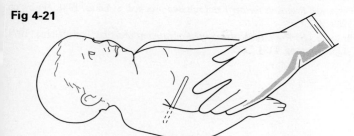

12. Record hourly the "patient temperature" and "air temperature" readings from the isolette control panel windows. Manually check and record axillary temperature every four hours.

13. Use tightly fitting portholes to enter the isolette for infant care. This maintains stable air temperature inside. Minimize porthole entrance by clustering activities of infant care.[1,3]

14. Teach the family how to use portholes. **NEVER LEAVE PORTHOLES OPEN.**

15. **NEVER TURN THE POWER OFF AND LEAVE AN INFANT INSIDE AN ISOLETTE.**
    Hypothermia occurs rapidly when the isolette is turned off, causing cold stress to the infant.

References

[1]Liebermon AB: *The preemie parent's handbook,* New York, 1984, Dutton, pp. 46-47.

[2]Whaley LF, Wong DL: *Nursing care of infants and children,* St Louis, 1979, Mosby, pp. 252-253,338.

[3]Korones SB: *High-risk newborn infants,* St Louis, 1986, Mosby, pp. 90-93.

[4]Perez RH: *Protocols for perinatal nursing practice,* St Louis, 1981, Mosby, pp. 259-265.

[5]Brunner LS: *The Lippincott manual of nursing practice,* Philadelphia, 1974, Lippincott, pp. 1124-1125.

Inserting Nasogastric (NG) and Orogastric (OG) Tubes

➤ **PURPOSE**

To correctly place a NG or OG tube for one of the following purposes:
- to decompress the stomach
- to lavage the stomach
- to instill medications
- to administer feedings

➤ **SUPPLIES**

Appropriate size NG tube
1/2" adhesive tape
Water-soluble lubricant
Nonsterile gloves
Goggles
Stethoscope
One 20 ml syringe
Functional suction apparatus
pH paper

➤ **PROCEDURE**

1. Determine the need for a NG or OG tube.
   Since infants < 6 months are obligate nose breathers, an OG is preferred in this age group.

2. Assemble supplies. Select the appropriate NG catheter for the child's size, as outlined in Table 4-1.
   Pediatric emergency tape may also be used to help select an appropriate size catheter.

Table 4-1 Sizes of NG Catheters by Pediatric Weight						
NG Size	5F	8F	10F	12F	14F	16F
Child's Weight	2 kg	3-9 kg	10-20 kg	20-30 kg	30-50 kg	50 kg+

From Skale N: *Manual of pediatric nursing procedures,* Philadelphia, 1992, Lippincott.

3. Procure assistance in restraining the child.

4. Prepare the child for the procedure.

- If the child is 2 to 7 years old, tell him or her immediately before the procedure and explain how it will feel.
- If the child is older, explain the procedure 5 to 10 minutes before starting it.

4. Explain the procedure and rationale to the parents.

5. Wash hands.

6. Put on goggles and gloves. Maintain universal precautions throughout the procedure.

7. Measure the length of the NG tube to be inserted by measuring from the nose to the earlobe and then to a point midway between the xyphoid process and the umbilicus[1,2,3]* (Fig. 4-22).

Fig 4-22

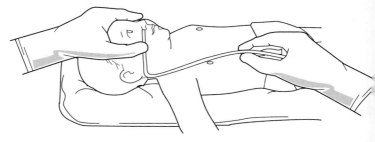

---

*Studies of measurement methods for proper NG/OG placement conclude that common measuring techniques are inaccurate and err by being too short.[1,4,5,6] Calculations based on the child's height predict esophageal length in children from 1 month to 4 years of age[4,5] [EL = 7.08 + (.216 × height)]; however, the optimal placement of the gastric tube beyond the esophageal length is undetermined. Ultimately confirm the gastric tube placement by x-ray.

8. Mark the tube with a piece of tape at this spot (Fig. 4-23).

Fig 4-23

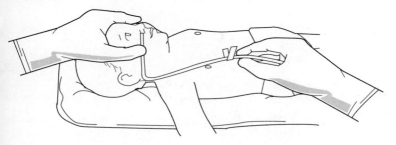

9. Lubricate the end of the gastric tube with water-soluble lubricant if inserting nasally (Fig. 4-24).

Fig 4-24

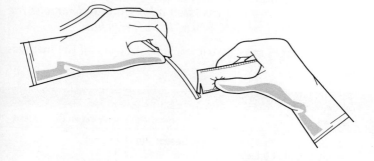

10. To insert the tube nasally, direct the tube along the floor of the nostril to the posterior pharyngeal wall and then firmly direct it downward (Fig. 4-25). To insert the tube orally, direct the tube to the back of the tongue and then firmly direct downward.

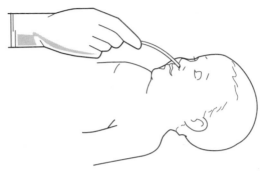

Fig 4-25

11. Continue advancing the tube until the tape mark is at the nostril or lip. Advance during inspiration, if possible.
If the tube meets resistance or if the child begins to vomit or has respiratory distress, stop advancing and remove the tube. The tube may be placed in the bronchus.

12. Check for correct gastric placement by one of the methods outlined in Table 4-2.[7,8]

Table 4-2 Gastric Placement of NG and OG Tubes	
Method	**Confirmation of Gastric Placement**
Aspirate gastric fluid from distal end of tube. Inject approximately 5 ml of air into the tube and auscultate with a stethoscope over the stomach area.	Gastric fluid can be aspirated. A pH ≤ 3 indicates gastric content. A "swoosh" or a "burp" can be heard over the stomach area.

13. Secure the tube according to "Securing Nasogastric (NG) and Orogastric (OG) Tubes."

14. Label the tube with your initials, the date, and time.

15. Give the child positive feedback.

References

[1]Weibley TT et al: Gavage tube insertion in the premature infant, *MCN Am J Matern Child Nurs* 12(1):24-27, 1987.

[2]Clemence B: Procedures involving the gastrointestinal and genitourinary systems. In Bernardo LM, Bove M, eds.: *Pediatric emergency procedures,* Boston, 1993, Jones & Bartlett, pp. 125-142.

[3]Skale N: Nasogastric insertion. In *Manual of pediatric nursing procedures,* Philadelphia, 1992, Lippincott, pp. 406-409.

[4]Ellett M et al: Predicting the distance for gavage tube placement in children, *Pediatr Nurs* 18(2):119-123, 127, 1992.

[5]Beckstrand J et al: The distance to the stomach for feeding tube placement in children predicted from regression on height, *Res in Nurs Health* 13(6):411-420, 1990.

[6]Lynn MR: Gastric tube insertion length:routine or researchable? *J Pediatr Nurs* 6(2):127-128, 1991.

[7]Comp D, Otten N: How to insert and remove nasogastric tubes quickly and easily, *Nursing 90* 90(9):59-64, 1990.

[8]Walsh SM, Banks LA: How to insert a small-bore feeding tube safely, *Nursing 90* 90(3):55-59, 1990.

Securing Nasogastric (NG) and Orogastric (OG) Tubes

➤ **PURPOSE**

To adequately secure a NG or OG tube and prevent it from being dislodged.

➤ **SUPPLIES**

¹/₄″ to ¹/₂″ adhesive tape

➤ **PROCEDURE—Nasogastric Tube**

1. Place a piece of tape (1 cm × 10 cm), adhesive side up, under the NG tube immediately beneath the nostril. Wrap it around the NG tube and extend the ends across the cheek and under the nose[1] (Fig. 4-26).
   Securing the NG tube beneath the nostril instead of to the nostril prevents possible sores on the nostril.

Fig 4-26

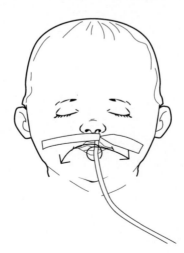

2. Secure the NG tube on the cheek with another piece of tape (1 cm × 5 cm) (Fig. 4-27).

Fig 4-27

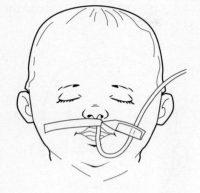

3. Fold a piece of tape (2 cm × 5 cm) over the NG tube approximately 15 to 20 cm from the nostril. Use a safety pin to secure the tape to the child's gown (Fig. 4-28).

Fig 4-28

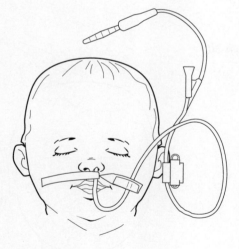

➤ **PROCEDURE—*Orogastric Tube***

1. Place a piece of tape (1 cm × 10 cm), adhesive side up, under the OG tube immediately outside the corner of the mouth. Wrap it around the OG tube and extend the ends across the cheek (Fig. 4-29).

Fig 4-29

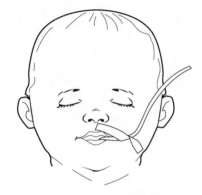

2. Continue with Steps 2 and 3 under "Nasogastric Tube" (Fig. 4-30).

Fig 4-30

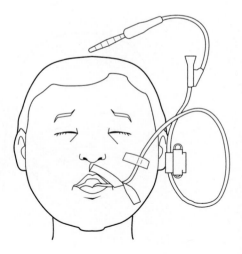

References

[1]Clemence B: Procedures involving the gastrointestinal and genitourinary systems. In Bernardo LM, Bove M, eds.: *Pediatric emergency procedures,* Boston, 1993, Jones & Bartlett, pp. 125-142.

Placing an Indwelling Urinary Catheter

➤ **PURPOSE**

To place an indwelling urinary catheter in order to relieve urinary retention, measure urinary output, or obtain a sterile urine specimen.

➤ **SUPPLIES**

Sterile catheterization kit **or**

Protective drape
Sterile gloves
Catheter of the appropriate size
Water-soluble lubricant
Forceps
10 ml syringe
Cotton balls or gauze
Povidone-iodine solution
Drainage set
Light source

➤ **PROCEDURE**

1. Determine the need for placement of an indwelling urinary catheter.
   Bladder catheterization is contraindicated in cases of suspected urinary trauma as evidenced by blood at the urethral meatus or perineal hematoma.[1,2]

2. Assemble supplies at the child's bedside. Select the appropriate catheter for the child's age, as shown in Table 4-3.
   The pediatric emergency tape may also be used to select an appropriate size catheter.

Table 4-3	Urinary Catheters
Age	**Size**
Newborn	5 to 8 F feeding tube
6 mo to 1 yr	5 to 8 F catheter
1 to 3 yr	10 F catheter
4 to 7 yr	10 to 12 F catheter
8 to 10 yr	12 F catheter
10 yr and up	14 F catheter

From Clemence B: Procedures involving the gastrointestinal and genitourinary systems. In Bernardo LM, Bove M, eds.: *Pediatric emergency nursing procedures*, Boston, 1993, Jones & Bartlett; Aoki BY, McCloskey K: *Evaluation, stabilization, and transport of the critically ill child*, St Louis, 1992, Mosby.

3. Seek assistance from another health care provider to ensure proper positioning of the child during the procedure.

4. Explain to the child and the family the need for bladder catheterization.

5. Provide privacy.

6. Wash hands and put on gloves. Maintain universal precautions throughout the entire procedure.

7. Place the infant or the child in a supine position. Place a female infant or child in a frogleg position.

8. Position lighting for adequate illumination of the urinary meatus.

9. Open the catheterization kit or assembled equipment using sterile technique.

10. Put on sterile gloves and arrange equipment for easy access during procedure. Test the balloon of the indwelling catheter by inflating and deflating. Observe for leaks.

11. Place drapes around the meatal opening.

12. Cleanse the meatal area:

- Female
  Separate the labia minor and identify the meatus. Using povidone-iodine soaked cotton balls and forceps, cleanse first down the middle, then down each side from the meatus to the rectum.[1]

- Male
  If necessary, retract the foreskin; lift the penis perpendicular to the body. Using a circular motion, cleanse from the meatal opening around the penis with povidone-iodine soaked cotton balls and forceps.[1]

13. Lubricate the insertion tip of the catheter.

14. Slowly insert the catheter into the urinary meatus until urine is obtained (Figs. 4-31 and 4-32). If resistance or obstruction is met, remove the catheter. Attempt placement a second time with a smaller catheter.

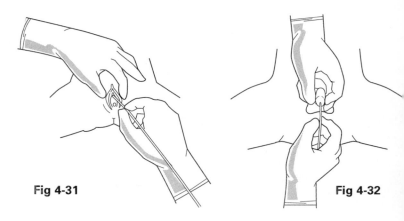

Fig 4-31

Fig 4-32

15. Inflate the balloon of the indwelling catheter with sterile water or saline in the amount indicated on the catheter or package.

16. Attach the urinary drainage bag to the catheter. Obtain a specimen if needed. Keep the drainage bag below bladder level at all times.[3]

17. Gently tug on the catheter. If the balloon is properly inflated, it will resist movement.[3]

18. Document the time of catheterization, size of the catheter, the amount, color and odor of urine obtained, and how the child tolerated the procedure.

19. Give the child positive feedback.

References

[1]Clemence B: Procedures involving the gastrointestinal and genitourinary systems. In Bernardo LM, Bove M, eds.: *Pediatric emergency nursing procedures*, Boston, 1993, Jones & Bartlett, 139-141.

[2]Aoki BY, McCloskey K: *Evaluation, stabilization, and transport of the critically ill child,* Mosby, 1992, p. 279.

[3]Earnest VV: *Clinical skills in nursing practice*, ed 2, Philadelphia, 1993, Lippincott, pp.592-612.

Securing an Indwelling Urinary Catheter

➤ *PURPOSE*

To secure an indwelling catheter to prevent accidental dislodgment and discomfort caused by pulling on the internal sphincter.[1]

➤ *SUPPLIES*

Nonsterile gloves
1/2″ adhesive tape

➤ *PROCEDURE*

• Female

Anchor the catheter to the medial aspect of either thigh using a piece of tape (1/2" × 3"). Allow for some "slack" when securing (Fig. 4-33).

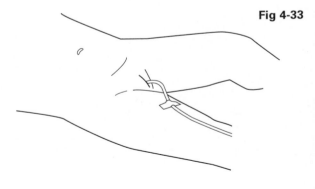

Fig 4-33

- **Male**

  Anchor the catheter to lower quadrant of the abdomen or thigh using a piece of tape (½" × 3"). This method will eliminate pressure and irritation on the underside of the penis and prevent a urethral stricture (Figs. 4-34 and 4-35).[1,2]

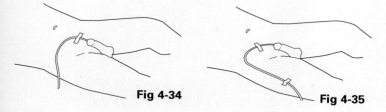

Fig 4-34   **Fig 4-35**

References

[1]Lewis L, Timby BK: *Fundamental skills and concepts in patient care,* ed 4, Philadelphia, 1988, Lippincott, pp. 592-612.

[2]Wieck L, King E, Dyer M: *Illustrated manual of nursing techniques,* ed 3, Philadelphia, 1986, Lippincott, pp. 271.

CHAPTER

5

Developmental Issues

Care of the Newborn (up to 1 month)

➤ **PURPOSE**

To describe normal newborn behavior and adapt interventions to developmental level.

➤ **SOCIAL SKILLS**

- cries
- responds similarly to family and strangers
- attends to a variety of sounds

➤ **MOTOR SKILLS**

- lifts head from prone position
- turns head from side to side
- coordinates suck, swallow, and respiration

➤ **NURSING INTERVENTIONS**

1. Keep the newborn covered or provide warming measures.

2. Talk to the newborn in a calm, soothing voice.

3. Offer the newborn a pacifier; sucking is a coping behavior for the newborn.

4. Observe before touching to obtain an accurate assessment.

5. Be sure hands are warm when touching the newborn.

6. Begin physical exam with the chest and abdomen. If the newborn begins to cry, examination of the chest or abdomen may be impossible.

7. Swaddle the newborn when the exam is complete.

➤ *ANTICIPATORY GUIDANCE*

1. Teach parents basic life support techniques, including measures for dealing with foreign body aspiration.

2. Ask parents if they have an infant (0 to 20 lbs.) car seat and reinforce the importance of placing the infant car seat in the back seat facing the rear. Reinforce proper techniques for belting the newborn into the seat and the seat into the car.

3. Counsel the parents on the importance of having a smoke detector on every floor of the home.

4. Inform parents of crib safety features.

5. Inform parents that the American Academy of Pediatrics now recommends *not* placing the infant prone to sleep in an attempt to reduce the incidence of sudden infant death syndrome (SIDS).

6. Teach parents to never leave their infant (or child) locked in a car.

References

Conway AE: Psychosocial considerations for the child and family. In Bernardo LM, Bove M, eds.: *Pediatric emergency nursing procedures,* Boston, 1993, Jones & Bartlett, pp. 11-27.

Dierking B, Reynolds EA, Ramenofsky ML: The stress of trauma, *JEMS* 50-52, 1988.

Gaynard L et al: Talking with children and families about health care experiences. In *Psychological care of children in hospitals: a clinical practice manual from the ACCH Child Life Research Project,* Bethesda, Md., 1990, Association for the Care of Children's Health, pp. 57-65.

Hazinski MF et al: Pediatric injury prevention, *Ann Emerg Med* 22(2, part 2):456-467, 1993.

Nass R: Rapid assessment of mental status in the infant and young child, *Emerg Med Clin North Am* 5(4):739-750, 1987.

Norwood SS: Dealing with children and families. In Norwood SS, Zaritsky AL, eds.: *Guidelines for pediatric emergency care,* 1992, North Carolina Emergency Medical Services for Children Project.

Skale N: *Manual of nursing procedures,* Philadelphia, 1992, Lippincott.

Widner-Kolberg MR: The nurse's role in pediatric injury prevention, *Crit Care Nurs Clinics North Am* 3(3):391-397, 1991.

Winn DG, Agran PF, Castillo DN: Pedestrian injuries to children younger than five years of age, *Pediatrics* 88:776-782, 1991.

Woolf A et al.: Prevention of childhood poisoning: efficacy of an educational program carried out in an emergency clinic, *Pediatrics* 80:359-363, 1987.

Care of the Infant
(1 to 12 months)

➤ **PURPOSE**

To describe normal infant behavior and adapt interventions to developmental level.

➤ **SOCIAL SKILLS**

- smiles and laughs out loud
- language ranges from single sounds (5 to 6 months) to 2 to 5 words with meaning (12 months)
- understands and responds to "No"
- responds to own name
- begins to recognize and act shy or fearful around strangers (5 to 6 months)
- very sensitive to physical environment

➤ **MOTOR SKILLS**

- sucking still a major coping mechanism
- explores environment by mouthing objects
- enjoys unrestricted movement
- grasps objects (4 to 5 months)
- rolls from stomach to back and from back to stomach (5 to 8 months)
- sits alone (7 to 9 months)
- crawls everywhere very quickly (10 to 12 months)
- stands alone and may be walking alone

➤ **NURSING INTERVENTIONS**

1. Keep the infant covered or provide warming measures.

2. Involve parents in the care of their infant as much as possible.

3. Assess the infant in parent's arms or lap if possible. Approach the infant at his or her physical level.

4. Develop rapport by cooing, tickling, and peek-a-boo games, but still keep parents close by.

5. Offer the infant a pacifier if parents approve.

6. Observe before touching to obtain an accurate assessment.

7. Be sure hands and equipment are warm when examining the infant.

8. Begin exam with the chest and abdomen.

9. Be careful not to leave small objects within the infant's reach.

10. Be careful not to leave the infant unsupervised on the exam table even momentarily.

11. Refrain from immobilizing the hand that the infant prefers to suck.

12. Allow rest periods between procedures.

➤ *ANTICIPATORY GUIDANCE*

1. Teach parents basic life support techniques, including measures for foreign body aspiration.

2. Teach parents to remove from the infant's environment small objects such as peanuts, coins, or buttons.

3. Teach parents the importance of removing all household cleaners and medicines from the infant's environment, including containers kept in the garage.

4. Give parents a phone number sticker for the Poison Control Center.

5. Counsel parents to use syrup of ipecac only as advised by the Poison Control Center.

6. Teach parents to avoid giving the infant balloons to play with.

7. Encourage parents to never leave the infant alone on the changing table.

8. Counsel parents on placing the infant in a playpen or high chair when cooking.

9. Teach parents the importance of gates on all stairs in the home.

10. Teach parents the importance of keeping chairs away from the table, counters, and windows, as infants will use chairs to climb onto other surfaces.

11. Counsel parents on the importance of lowering the water temperature below 120° C.

12. Counsel parents on the importance of *never* leaving the infant alone in the bathtub, even for the time it takes to answer the phone.

13. For parents with residential swimming pools, give literature on the laws regarding fences around the pool if applicable in your region.
    A 5-foot-high fence that completely surrounds the pool and has a self-closing and self-latching gate is recommended.

14. Inform parents of the importance of a toddler car seat and reinforce proper procedures for belting the infant and the seat.

15. Teach parents the importance of using outlet plugs to prevent infants from putting objects into the outlet.

16. Encourage parents to use stationary walking agents instead of walkers for infants.

References

Conway AE: Psychosocial considerations for the child and family. In Bernardo LM, Bove M, eds.: *Pediatric emergency nursing procedures,* Boston, 1993, Jones & Bartlett, pp. 11-27.

Dierking B, Reynolds EA, Ramenofsky ML: The stress of trauma, *JEMS* 50-52, 1988.

Gaynard L et al: Talking with children and families about health care experiences. In *Psychological care of children in hospitals: a clinical practice manual from the ACCH Child Life Research Project,* Bethesda, Md., 1990, Association for the Care of Children's Health, pp. 57-65.

Hazinski MF et al: Pediatric injury prevention, *Ann Emerg Med* 22(2 part 2):456-467, 1993.

Nass R: Rapid assessment of mental status in the infant and young child, *Emerg Med Clin North Am* 5(4):739-750, 1987.

Norwood SS: Dealing with children and families. In Norwood SS, Zaritsky AL, eds.: *Guidelines for pediatric emergency care*, 1992, North Carolina Emergency Medical Services for Children Project.

Skale N: *Manual of nursing procedures*, Philadelphia, 1992, Lippincott.

Widner-Kolberg MR: The nurse's role in pediatric injury prevention, *Crit Care Nurs Clinics North Am* 3(3):391-397, 1991.

Winn DG, Agran PF, Castillo DN: Pedestrian injuries to children younger than five years of age, *Pediatrics* 88:776-782, 1991.

Woolf A et al: Prevention of childhood poisoning: efficacy of an educational program carried out in an emergency clinic, *Pediatrics* 80:359-363, 1987.

Care of the Toddler (1 to 3 years)

➤ **PURPOSE**

To describe normal toddler behavior and adapt interventions to developmental level.

➤ **SOCIAL SKILLS**

- wants to do things for self
- likes to help
- curious about environment and enjoys independence
- asks questions
- has short attention span
- fears parents leaving
- can express several intelligible words (18 months)
- progresses to 2 to 3 word phrases (2 years)
- understands more language than is able to express
- may understand language, but is unlikely to believe reassurances
- starts to develop memory for things and events
- has poor understanding of time
- does not fully understand cause and effect
- blames the cause of illness or injury on something completely unrelated; "magical thinking"
- may think that he or she has caused the illness or injury
- may cope with fear by regressing or being aggressive

➤ **MOTOR SKILLS**

- increased mobility (runs, jumps, rides toys)
- walks up stairs (18 months)
- can scribble spontaneously (2 to 3 years)

➤ NURSING INTERVENTIONS

1. Involve the parents as much as possible.

2. Keep parents nearby if they cannot be involved.

3. Approach the toddler slowly so as not to frighten him or her.

4. Bend down, sit, or squat to be on the toddler's eye level.

5. Begin exam with the trunk.

6. Limit exam to the bare essentials.

7. Explain procedures immediately before they will begin.

8. Use simple, concrete terms when explaining procedures.

9. Explain procedures by how they will feel, not by why they must be done.

10. Give the toddler choices, but only choices that exist.

11. Reassure the toddler that it is all right to cry but not to kick, bite, or hit.

12. Allow him or her as much movement as possible; for instance, if restraining one extremity, give permission to move another.

13. Reassure the toddler that he or she is not being punished.

14. Observe for pain behaviors.

15. Use distraction techniques if the toddler becomes anxious, then proceed as quickly as possible.

16. Provide positive feedback after the procedure.

17. Give a sticker or small toy as a reward.

➤ ANTICIPATORY GUIDANCE

1. Reinforce the importance of a toddler car seat and proper procedure for belting the toddler and the seat.

2. Reinforce the importance of gates on all stairs in the home.

3. Teach parents the importance of a fenced-in play area for the toddler.

4. Encourage parents to always hold the toddler's hand when crossing the street.

5. Reinforce the importance of keeping chairs away from the table, counters, and windows.

6. Reinforce the importance of removing all household cleaners and medicines from the toddler's environment, including containers kept in the garage. Child-proof devices do not replace removing poisonous substances.

7. Make sure parents have phone number sticker for the Poison Control Center.

8. Reinforce using syrup of ipecac only with instructions from the Poison Control Center.

9. For parents with residential swimming pools, give literature on the laws regarding fences around the pool if applicable in your region.
   A 5-foot-high fence that completely surrounds the pool and has a self-closing and self-latching gate is recommended.

10. Reinforce with parents the importance of using outlet plugs to prevent toddlers from putting objects into the outlet.

11. Encourage parents to use caution with hot items.

   • Place the iron and cord out of the toddler's reach.
   • Place hot cups of coffee or hot pans away from the edge of the counter.
   • Turn handles of cooking pots inward on the stovetop.

References

Conway AE: Psychosocial considerations for the child and family. In Bernardo LM, Bove M, eds.: *Pediatric emergency nursing procedures*, Boston, 1993, Jones & Bartlett, pp. 11-27.

Dierking B, Reynolds EA, Ramenofsky ML: The stress of trauma, *JEMS* 50-52, 1988.

Gaynard L et al: Talking with children and families about health care experiences. In *Psychological care of children in hospitals: a clinical practice manual from the ACCH Child Life Research Project*, Bethesda, Md., 1990, Association for the Care of Children's Health, pp. 57-65.

Hazinski MF et al: Pediatric injury prevention, *Ann Emerg Med* 22(2 part 2):456-467, 1993.

Nass R: Rapid assessment of mental status in the infant and young child, *Emerg Med Clin North Am* 5(4):739-750, 1987.

Norwood SS: Dealing with children and families. In Norwood SS, Zaritsky AL, eds.: *Guidelines for pediatric emergency care*, 1992, North Carolina Emergency Medical Services for Children Project.

Reynolds EA, Ramenofsky ML: The emotional impact of trauma on toddlers, *MCN Am J Matern Child Nurs* 13:106-109, 1988.

Skale N: *Manual of nursing procedures*, Philadelphia, 1992, Lippincott.

Widner-Kolberg MR: The nurse's role in pediatric injury prevention, *Crit Care Nurs Clinics North Am* 3(3):391-397, 1991.

Winn DG, Agran PF, Castillo DN: Pedestrian injuries to children younger than five years of age, *Pediatrics* 88:776-782, 1991.

Woolf A et al: Prevention of childhood poisoning: efficacy of an educational program carried out in an emergency clinic, *Pediatrics* 80:359-363, 1987.

Care of the Preschooler
(3 to 5 years)

➤ *PURPOSE*

To describe normal preschooler behavior and adapt interventions to developmental level.

➤ *SOCIAL SKILLS*

- likes to help
- frequently resorts to "I don't know"
- fears bodily injury
- may tolerate brief separations from parents if given explanations
- can use language to express thoughts and feelings and to describe experiences
- may have an imaginary friend
- may talk and ask questions constantly
- still deals in "magical thinking"; hard to distinguish between make-believe and reality
- still does not fully understand cause and effect
- has developed a strong, simplistic sense of right and wrong
- has limited understanding of death

➤ *MOTOR SKILLS*

- continues to explore with curiosity
- can draw pictures and some letters
- likes to play games
- can climb a ladder
- may ride 2-wheel bike
- hops, skips, and jumps

➤ NURSING INTERVENTIONS

1. Examine with parents present.

2. Limit exam if possible; preschoolers are modest.

3. Replace one item of clothing before taking off another.

4. Explain a procedure shortly before it will happen.

5. Explain procedures in simple, concrete terms.

6. Explain procedures by how they feel.

7. Use caution when using medical terms, as they might have a different meaning for the preschooler. Explain medical terms with an example that is familiar to the preschooler.

8. Use a doll or stuffed animal when explaining procedures.

9. Allow him or her to handle the equipment if appropriate.

10. Offer the preschooler choices when appropriate.

11. Use pronouns accurately. If you mean "you," do not use "us" or "we."

12. Ask the preschooler what he or she understands about what is happening.

13. Encourage the preschooler to verbalize potential fears. Ask about previous hospital experiences.

14. Reassure the preschooler that he or she is not being punished.

15. Offer abundant reassurances.

16. Observe for masked pain behaviors.

17. Reward the preschooler with stickers.

18. Use bandages liberally. Looking at an injury increases the preschooler's anxiety.

➤ ANTICIPATORY GUIDANCE

1. Encourage parents not to let their preschooler ride a bicycle in the street.

2. Teach the preschooler the importance of wearing a helmet when riding his or her bicycle.

3. Encourage parents to hold their preschooler's hand when crossing the street.

4. Reinforce with the preschooler the importance of wearing a safety belt at all times in the car.

5. Teach the preschooler not to take things from or go with a stranger.

6. Teach the preschooler not to go near a pond, creek, or other body of water without an adult.

7. Emphasize to the preschooler that he or she should *never* touch a gun and should get an adult if he or she sees one.

8. Continue teaching parents to remove all household cleaners and medicines from the preschooler's environment, including environments away from home such as grandparents' or other relatives' homes.

References

Conway AE: Psychosocial considerations for the child and family. In Bernardo LM, Bove M, eds.: *Pediatric emergency nursing procedures,* Boston, 1993, Jones & Bartlett, pp. 11-27.

Dierking B, Reynolds EA, Ramenofsky ML: The stress of trauma, *JEMS* 50-52, 1988.

Gaynard L: Talking with children and families about health care experiences. In *Psychological care of children in hospitals: a clinical practice manual from the ACCH Child Life Research Project,* Bethesda, Md., 1990, Association for the Care of Children's Health, pp. 57-65.

Hazinski MF: Pediatric injury prevention, *Ann Emerg Med* 22(2 part 2):456-467, 1993.

Nass R: Rapid assessment of mental status in the infant and young child, *Emerg Med Clin North Am* 5(4):739-750, 1987.

Norwood SS: Dealing with children and families. In Norwood SS, Zaritsky AL, eds.: *Guidelines for Pediatric Emergency Care,,* 1992, North Carolina Emergency Medical Services for Children Project.

Skale N: *Manual of nursing procedures,* Philadelphia, 1992, Lippincott.

Widner-Kolberg MR: The nurse's role in pediatric injury prevention, *Crit Care Nurs Clinics North Am* 3(3):391-397, 1991.

Winn DG, Agran PF, Castillo DN: Pedestrian injuries to children younger than five years of age, *Pediatrics* 88:776-782, 1991.

Woolf A et al.: Prevention of childhood poisoning: efficacy of an educational program carried out in an emergency clinic, *Pediatrics* 80:359-363, 1987.

Care of the School-Age Child (5 to 12 years)

PURPOSE

To describe normal school-age behavior and adapt interventions to developmental level.

SOCIAL SKILLS

- usually cooperative
- values peers
- enjoys structure and rules
- often is modest
- concerned about body integrity
- interested in his or her body
- very sensitive to surroundings
- possesses an expanding vocabulary and increased understanding of concepts
- able to describe location and duration of pain
- understands cause and effect with concrete examples
- views illness as happening because of "contamination" with something bad, for instance "germs"
- still obsessed with fairness
- aware of and afraid of death

MOTOR SKILLS

- has fine motor hand control
- plays and works hard
- may be involved in organized sports

➤ *NURSING INTERVENTIONS*

1. Maintain privacy.

2. Allow the parents to be present; encourage parents to help the child cope.

3. Obtain a history from the child as well as from the parents.

4. Encourage the child to participate in his or her care.

5. Avoid letting the child view other procedures or events occurring in the emergency department.

6. Allow time for the child to ask questions when explaining procedure.

7. Explain procedures with anatomical models or pictures and equipment.

8. Offer choices.

9. Ask the child what he or she understands about what is happening.

10. Reassure the child that he or she is not being punished.

11. Observe for masked pain behaviors.

12. Offer abundant reassurances throughout the procedure.

➤ *ANTICIPATORY GUIDANCE*

1. Teach the child safety rules of the street.

2. Teach the child safety rules on the bicycle.

3. Encourage the child not to ride his or her bicycle on the street.

4. Reinforce to the child the importance of wearing a helmet.

5. Provide parents with literature on helmets.

6. Reinforce with the child the importance of wearing a seat belt every time he or she rides in a car.

7. Counsel parents to continue to supervise children when they are playing outside.

8. Encourage the child to wear a helmet and skin pads while playing sports.

9. Discuss with the child the harmful side effects of illicit drugs.

10. Discuss with the child alternative strategies for violent behavior, such as not using guns and knives.

11. Counsel parents to discuss potential peer pressure issues with their child, such as use of illicit drugs, use of guns and knives, and sexual activity.

12. Educate parents regarding the physical, physiological, and emotional changes of puberty.

References

Conway AE: Psychosocial considerations for the child and family. In Bernardo LM, Bove M, eds.: *Pediatric emergency nursing procedures,* Boston, 1993, Jones & Bartlett, pp. 11-27.

Dierking B, Reynolds EA, Ramenofsky ML: The stress of trauma, *JEMS* 50-52, 1988.

Gaynard L: Talking with children and families about health care experiences. In *Psychological care of children in hospitals: a clinical practice manual from the ACCH Child Life Research Project,* Bethesda, Md., 1990, Association for the Care of Children's Health, pp. 57-65.

Hazinski MF et al: Pediatric injury prevention, *Ann Emerg Med* 22(2 part 2):456-467, 1993.

Nass R: Rapid assessment of mental status in the infant and young child, *Emerg Med Clin North Am* 5(4):739-750, 1987.

Norwood SS: Dealing with children and families. In Norwood SS, Zaritsky AL, eds.: *Guidelines for pediatric emergency care,* 1992, North Carolina Emergency Medical Services for Children Project.

Skale N: *Manual of nursing procedures,* Philadelphia, 1992, Lippincott.

Widner-Kolberg MR: The nurse's role in pediatric injury prevention, *Crit Care Nurs Clinics North Am* 3(3):391-397, 1991.

Winn DG, Agran PF, Castillo DN: Pedestrian injuries to children younger than five years of age, *Pediatrics* 88:776-782, 1991.

Woolf A et al: Prevention of childhood poisoning: efficacy of an educational program carried out in an emergency clinic, *Pediatrics* 80:359-363, 1987.

Care of the Adolescent
(12 to 18 years)

➤ **PURPOSE**

To describe normal adolescent behavior and adapt inter
ventions to developmental level.

➤ **SOCIAL SKILLS**

- very involved with peer group
- influenced by peer pressure
- may have hostility toward parents
- interested in opposite sex
- self-conscious about body image
- very critical of his or her own appearance and behaviors
- beginning to understand anatomy and physiology of
  own body
- possesses ability for abstract thought
- can understand cause and effect
- still has many fears
- views death realistically

➤ **MOTOR SKILLS**

- often awkward and uncoordinated
- physically active but tires easily

➤ **NURSING INTERVENTIONS**

1. Talk to the adolescent before talking with parents.

2. Ask the adolescent if he or she prefers to have parents present

3. Provide measures for privacy. Use gowns and drapes.

4. Approach in adult fashion, but offer abundant reassurances.

5. Allow ample time before the procedure for explanations.

6. Explain procedures thoroughly.

7. Incorporate the adolescent in decision making regarding his or her treatment.

8. Encourage him or her to verbalize feelings.

9. Observe for masked pain behaviors.

➤ *ANTICIPATORY GUIDELINES*

1. Reinforce with the adolescent the importance of wearing a seat belt every time he or she rides in a car or is the driver.

2. Discuss with the adolescent the danger of drinking and driving or drinking with any activity such as boating, skiing, or hunting.

3. Discuss with the adolescent the harmful side effects of illicit drugs.

4. Encourage the adolescent to practice safe sex if sexually active.

References

Conway AE: Psychosocial considerations for the child and family. In Bernardo LM, Bove M, eds.: *Pediatric emergency nursing procedures,* Boston, 1993, Jones & Bartlett, pp. 11-27.

Dierking B, Reynolds EA, Ramenofsky ML: The stress of trauma, *JEMS* 50-52, 1988.

Gaynard L et al: Talking with children and families about health care experiences. In *Psychological care of children in hospitals: a clinical practice manual from the ACCH Child Life Research Project,* Bethesda, Md., 1990, Association for the Care of Children's Health, pp. 57-65.

Hazinski MF et al: Pediatric injury prevention, *Ann Emerg Med* 22(2 part 2):456-467, 1993.

Nass R: Rapid assessment of mental status in the infant and young child, *Emerg Med Clin North Am* 5(4):739-750, 1987.

Norwood SS: Dealing with children and families. In Norwood SS, Zaritsky AL, eds.: *Guidelines for pediatric emergency care,* 1992, North Carolina Emergency Medical Services for Children Project.

Skale N: *Manual of nursing procedures,* Philadelphia, 1992, Lippincott.

Widner-Kolberg MR: The nurse's role in pediatric injury prevention, *Crit Care Nurs Clinics North Am* 3(3):391-397, 1991.

Winn DG, Agran PF, Castillo DN: Pedestrian injuries to children younger than five years of age, *Pediatrics* 88:776-782, 1991.

Woolf A et al: Prevention of childhood poisoning: efficacy of an educational program carried out in an emergency clinic, *Pediatrics,* 80:359-363, 1987.

CHAPTER

6

Case Studies

Case Study 1

◆ You receive in your emergency department (ED) a 4-year-old male with a history of hydrocephalus s/p a VP shunt placement shortly after birth. Mother reports that the child woke up this AM with a high fever and she has been unable to bring it down with acetaminophen.

Objective assessment reveals a lethargic boy who responds to speech but is content to lie quietly on the exam bed. Estimated weight by the pediatric emergency tape is 13 kg.

HR = 150 beats/minute   RR = 24 breaths/minute
T = 39.5° C rectally (You cannot locate a blood pressure cuff in the right size and therefore are unable to obtain a blood pressure reading.)

1. What is your first priority?

◆ The child's airway is uncompromised and he is breathing without effort at 24 breaths/minute. No retractions or nasal flaring noted. Breath sounds are clear and equal bilaterally, decreased in bases.

Apical heart rate is strong and regular at 150 beats/minute; S_1 and S_2 present without murmur. Extremities are pink and hot with 2 second capillary refill. Peripheral pulses are +2 in all four extremities.

As part of a sepsis workup, the physician requests blood cultures, CBC with differential, serum electrolytes, and an IV.

2. Where is the best place to draw blood in this child?

3. How do you explain to the child what you will be doing?

4. Your ED stocks butterfly needles in sizes 25 and 23 gauge. Which do you use?

5. If your ED does not stock butterfly needles, what do you use?

6. Where do you start an IV in this child?

7. What size over-the-needle catheter do you use to start an IV in this child?

8. Once you obtain a flashback, what maneuver will enhance threading of the catheter?

◆ You successfully start a 20 gauge IV in his left hand. You were unable to draw blood samples with the IV start, however, so you obtained the samples from the right antecubital fossa.

9. How do you secure the IV in his left hand?

10. The resident orders maintenance fluids of $D_5 \frac{1}{4} NS$ at 46 ml/hour. Is this an appropriate maintenance fluid and rate for this child?

◆ The resident orders acetaminophen suppository 200 mg now, ceftriaxone 600 mg IV q12 hrs, and vancomycin 130 mg IV q8 hrs. Your unit secretary informs you that the radiology department is ready for a chest film and has requested that you send the child immediately.

11. What do you do?

12. How do you check the dose of ceftriaxone?

13. How do you check the dose of vancomycin?

◆ According to your pediatric reference manual, this amount of vancomycin must be diluted in at least 26 ml and given over at least 60 minutes. After the ceftriaxone is in, you start the vancomycin on a syringe pump.

The child remains stable, so you prepare him for transport to radiology and then to the pediatric intensive care unit (PICU).

SUGGESTED ANSWERS

1. As with any admission, start with the ABCs.
    a. Airway—Ensure that the airway is patent and stable. If necessary, open the airway and suction any obvious secretions.
    b. Breathing—After the airway is secured, assess for adequate ventilation. Assess respiratory rate and effort by observing the child's face, neck, and chest. Look for retractions, nasal flaring, and anxiety. Note child's preferred position. Auscultate for breath sounds along the mid-axillary line. Observe skin color.
    c. Circulation—After the airway is established and adequate ventilation is obtained, assess the circulatory status. Assess extremities for skin color, peripheral pulses, capillary refill, and temperature. Note the heart rate and blood pressure (if available).

2. The antecubital fossa veins are ideal for drawing blood samples (see "Blood Sample Collection"). Each child is different, however, and veins in the hand may also be used for this 4-year-old. Since this child has a chronic condition and probably has had multiple blood draws, his mother may be able to identify past successful sites.

3. Assuming this child has normal cognitive development, tell him right before you are ready to begin the procedure. Use simple, concrete terms. Focus on how the blood draw will feel, not why you are doing it. Be honest.

    EXAMPLE
    "Tommy, I need to get a little bit of blood from inside your arm. I'm going to get it right here. It's going to hurt when I start, but I'll try to do it really fast. It's okay for you to cry when I do it."

    Offer abundant reassurances after the blood draw is done. Offer a sticker or small toy as a reward for the child.

4. A 23 gauge is less likely to clot that a 25 gauge; veins in a 13 kg child should tolerate a 23 gauge needle.

5. A 23 or 25 gauge needle and syringe may also be used; see "Blood Sample Collection."

6. Again, the mother may be able to direct you to a previous

successful site. Use distal sites first. Veins in the dorsum of the hand or the antecubital fossa may be used. Avoid the dominant hand if possible.

NOTE: YOU MAY WANT TO TRY TO START AN IV BEFORE DRAWING BLOOD; IF YOU CANNULATE A LARGE VEIN, BLOOD SAMPLES MAY BE DRAWN AT THE SAME TIME THE IV IS STARTED, REQUIRING ONE LESS NEEDLE STICK.

7. A 22, 20, or 18 gauge catheter for children 1 to 12 years old may be used.

8. Once a flashback is obtained, advance the needle 1 to 3 mm further to ensure the catheter is inserted beyond the bevel. This prevents the catheter bevel from catching on the vein wall.

9. See "Securing IV Catheters."

10. The recommended maintenance IV fluid for children is $D_5^1/4NS$. Potassium may be added after urine output is established and the electrolyte panel is completed.

   The recommended maintenance fluid rate for a 13 kg child is calculated by:

   40 ml/hr for the first 10 kg plus
   2 ml/kg/hr for every kg over 10 kg

Therefore: 40 ml/hr + 6 ml/hr = 46 ml/hr

11. It is imperative that this child receive antibiotics without delay; this is first priority. Call radiology and coordinate a time that allows you to start the antibiotics first.

12. Use a pediatric pharmacology reference manual. From *The Harriet Lane Handbook,* the recommended maintenance dose for ceftriaxone is 100 mg/kg/24 hr divided q12 hr.

The recommended dose for this child (weight = 13 kg) is:

---

100 mg × 13 kg = 1300 mg

1300 mg ÷ 2 = 650 mg

Therefore the ordered dose of 600 mg is appropriate. Be sure to check the frequency ordered also, as the recommended dose of 650 mg is based on a BID schedule (and a total daily dose of 1300 mg).

See "Calculating Pediatric Doses."

13. Use a pediatric pharmacology reference manual. From *The Harriet Lane Handbook*, the recommended maintenance dose for vancomycin is 10/mg/kg/dose q8 hr.

Therefore the recommended dose for this child (weight = 13 kg) is:

10 mg × 13 kg = 130 mg

Therefore the ordered dose of 130 mg q8 hr is appropriate. Again, always check the frequency ordered as well.

See "Calculating Pediatric Doses."

SUMMARY POINTS

1. Drawing blood samples and starting IVs in children is often a difficult task. Selecting the most accessible site offers the greatest chance of success. The antecubital fossa is the site of choice for drawing blood samples. For children 3 years and older, veins in the dorsum of the hand or the antecubital fossa may be used for IV insertion.
   If the child has a chronic condition that has required numerous blood draws or IV insertions, the parents may be able to identify previous successful sites.

2. Although checking pediatric medication doses is time-consuming, *it is imperative.* The margin of error is small and the consequences may be great. Use a pediatric pharmacology reference manual and consult with the physician if the dose is inappropriate.

Case Study 2

◆ You receive in your ED a 3-year-old male who was the victim of a bedroom fire started by an electric heater. The local paramedic squad transported the child; transport time was 5 minutes.

The child's estimated weight by pediatric emergency tape is 18 kg. The child was orally intubated in the field. A 12 NG salem sump was placed in his right nare and a 16 gauge IO line was started in his right lower leg with lactated ringer's (LR) infusing via a pressure bag.

HR = 169 beats/minute
BP = 90/60 mm Hg
RR = 20 breaths/minute (manual bagging)
The child is estimated to have 95% second and third degree burns to his head, chest, abdomen, and arms and legs bilaterally. Facial edema is present; his eyelids are swollen shut.

1. What is your first priority?

◆ The child is intubated with a 4.0 mm ETT, taped securely. The respiratory therapist is performing manual bag-valve ventilation with 100% oxygen at a rate of 20 breaths/minute with a PEEP of 8 cm H_2O. Bilateral breath sounds are clear and equal. An ABG was drawn and sent.

Bilateral femoral pulses are faint but present. Bilateral carotid pulses are present and strong. You are unable to check capillary refill because of the extent of the burns. Apical heart rate is strong and regular. Blood pressure is stable at 90/60 mm Hg.

2. Why is it important that this child was intubated in the field?

3. What are the clinical signs and symptoms of inhalation injury?

4. What size ETT do you expect in this child?

5. How do you secure the ETT?

◆ The child is being bag-valve ventilated with 100% O_2; tidal volume is approximately 250 ml, rate is 20 breaths/minute, and the PEEP is set at 8 cm H_2O. The initial ABG displays inadequate ventilation and oxygenation: pH = 7.10, $PaCO_2$ = 98, PaO_2 = 63.

6. What are possible causes of this ABG and what do you do?

◆ Bilateral breath sounds are equal with inspiratory and expiratory wheezes. The ETT is taped securely at 12.5 cm at the lip.

You decide to suction to rule out the possibility of secretions blocking the airway.

7. What size catheter do you use?

8. How far do you insert the catheter?

◆ The ETT is suctioned for minimal white secretions.

The O_2 tubing is connected to the O_2 source. The resuscitator device is functional and the operator is delivering manual breaths as ordered. The pop-off valve is permanently depressed in this resuscitator device.

You increase tidal volume to 300 ml, rate to 25 breaths/minute, and the PEEP to 12 cm H_2O, assuming decreased lung compliance. The physician performs a bilateral chest escharotomy.

Repeat ABG: pH = 7.24, $PaCO_2$ = 52, PaO_2 = 94.

During your circulatory assessment, objective assessment reveals that his right lower leg is more edematous than his left.

9. What are potential complications of an intraosseous line?

10. You assume the IO line is infiltrated and so prepare to start a new IO line. What equipment do you assemble? What size IO needle do you use?

11. Where do you place the IO line?

12. How do you insert the IO line?

13. How do you secure the IO line?

14. How do you fluid resuscitate this child?

15. After resuscitation, how do you calculate this child's maintenance IV fluid requirements?

16. With the child's airway and breathing status stable and fluid resuscitation begun, you prepare to transport the child to a burn ICU. What other interventions do you consider as you await a bed status report?

17. What other clinical condition needs to be ruled out in this child and why?

18. How is this condition diagnosed?

19. What is the role of pulse oximetry?

SUGGESTED ANSWERS

1. As with any admission, start with the ABCs.

   a. Airway—Ensure that the airway is patent and stable. Check ETT placement by auscultating over the mid-axillary line. Since breath sounds are easily transmitted in the pediatric patient, listening over the top of the chest may be confusing. If an end-title CO_2 device is available, confirm placement with it as well. Check the security of the tape on the ETT. If necessary, suction any obvious secretions.

   b. Breathing—After the airway is secured, assess for adequate ventilation. Observe chest excursion. Auscultate for breath sounds along the mid-axillary line.

   c. Circulation—After the airway is established and adequate ventilation is obtained, assess the circulatory status. Assess extremities for peripheral pulses, capillary refill, and temperature. Note the heart rate and blood pressure (if available).

2. The child is at risk for inhalation burns because he was the victim of a fire in an enclosed space. These burns produce marked edema in the upper airway. The edema peaks 6 to 8 hours after exposure and would make intubation difficult at this time.

3. • Burns to the face and neck
   • Charred secretions from the nose and/or mouth
   • Lack of consciousness
   • Apnea
   • Labored respirations
   • Singed nasal hair

4. The child is intubated with a 4.0 mm ETT; although a 5.0 mm ETT is expected based on the child's age and weight, tracheal edema from smoke inhalation may necessitate a smaller ETT.

5. See "Securing an Endotracheal Tube (ETT)." If there are burns on the face, the ETT may need to be secured with tracheostomy ties around the whole head instead of with tape.

6. a. ETT not in correct position (right mainstem or esophageal placement).
      Check bilateral breath sounds again in the mid-axillary region and over the abdomen. Ensure that the tape is secure.
   b. Pneumothorax.
      Ensure that breath sounds are equal bilaterally. If a pneumothorax is suspected, perform a needle thoracotomy.
   c. Clogged or kinked ETT.
      Ensure that the tube is not kinked. Suction to clear the ETT of potential secretions.
   d. Oxygen (O_2) setup not connected to O_2 flow.
      Ensure that the tubing is connected to the O_2 source.
   e. Operator failure.
      Ensure that the person ventilating and oxygenating is delivering adequate tidal volume and rate.
   f. Resuscitator device failure.
      Ensure that the bag-valve device is functioning properly. The pop-off valve may need to be depressed to deliver adequate pressures in a child with increased airway resistance.
   g. Decreased lung compliance due to inhalation and circumferential burns to the chest.
      Increase rate to adequately ventilate. Increase tidal volume and PEEP to adequately oxygenate and ventilate. If chest expansion is limited, consider an escharotomy.

7. An 8 F will definitely fit through a 4.0 ETT; a 10 F might fit. To determine the catheter size from the ETT size, multiply the ETT size by 2.

8. Note the centimeter marking at the end of the ETT and add one centimeter for the adapter to get the depth of insertion for the catheter (see "Suctioning"). Inserting the catheter too far past the ETT can produce trauma to the tissue.

9. • Subcutaneous or subperiosteal infiltration
   • Osteomyelitis
   • Epiphyseal plate damage
   • Cellulitis

10. • Bone marrow needle, spinal needle, or a specific intraosseous needle; size 15 gauge
    • Nonsterile gloves
    • Povidone-iodine solution
    • IV extension tubing (2 to 3 inches)
    • Three-way stopcock
    • 60 ml syringe
    • IV infusion setup

11. Your options will depend on the character of the burns at potential sites.

    • Tibial tuberosity of other leg: 1 to 3 cm below the tibial tuberosity
    • Distal femur site: 2 to 3 cm above the external condyles
    • Medial malleolus site: proximal to the medial malleolus and posterior to the saphenous vein

    During the initial resuscitation the IO can be inserted through burned tissue if none of the sites are intact. Ideally this child needs 2 large bore IV or IO lines; the extent of his burns require fluid boluses in addition to large amounts of maintenance fluids.

12. See "Intraosseus (IO) Needle Insertion."

13. See "Securing an Intraosseus (IO) Needle." If the line is placed through a burn, using gauze and tape may be inappropriate.

14. This child requires massive fluid resuscitation, not only because of the extent of his burns (major thermal burn > 40% total body surface area [BSA]) but also because he is displaying signs of shock (femoral pulses are faint).

a. Deliver 20 ml/kg of LR until femoral pulses are strong and peripheral pulses present. See "Fluid Bolus Administration."
b. Calculate burn fluid replacement by using the Parkland Formula:

$$3 \text{ to } 4 \text{ ml} \times \% \text{ BSA burned} \times \text{wt(kg)} = \text{resuscitation volume (ml)}$$

Administer half of this volume in the first 8 hours after the burn injury and administer the second half over the next 16 hours.

Therefore:

$$3 \text{ ml} \times 95 \times 18 \text{ kg} = 5130 \text{ ml over 24 hours}$$
$$5130 \div 2 = 2565 \text{ ml over first 8 hours}$$
$$2565 \div 8 = 320 \text{ ml/hr}$$

Administer this fluid on an infusion pump. LR is the fluid of choice.

NOTE: THIS CALCULATION IS NOT FOR MAINTENANCE IV FLUID RATES; BURN VICTIMS REQUIRE LARGE VOLUMES OF FLUID IN ADDITION TO MAINTENANCE REQUIREMENTS.

As fluid resuscitation continues, tissue perfusion may be impaired due to the constriction of eschar (making palpation of peripheral pulses impossible). An escharotomy may be needed—a surgical incision through the eschar to allow edema to occur without impairing infusion.

15. See "Calculating Maintenance Intravenous (IV) Fluid Requirements." An hourly rate for this child is calculated by:

The fluid of choice for maintenance IV fluids is $D_5 1/4 NS$.

---

40 ml/hr for the first 10 kg plus
2 ml/hr for every kg over 10 kg

Therefore 40 ml/hr + 16 ml/hr = 56 ml/hr

---

16. a. Place an indwelling urinary catheter to monitor fluid resuscitation (see "Placing an Indwelling Urinary Catheter"). A 10 to 12 F urinary catheter is appropriate for a child this size. Urine output > 1 ml/hr is adequate. If

urine output falls to less than 1 ml/hr, the child needs more fluid. Also monitor the color of the urine.

b. Administer analgesic agents intravenously. Even though third degree burns have destroyed the nerve endings and are theoretically painless, most burns are a combination of full and partial thickness. Use morphine sulfate (0.1 to 0.2 mg/kg/dose q2 to 4 hr) or fentanyl (1 to 2 µg/kg/dose q1 hr).

c. Remove clothing and jewelry. If clothing adheres to skin, cut it off.

d. Maintain body temperature. Consider warmed IV fluids with massive fluid resuscitation. Also turn up the temperature in the room, if possible, and obtain an overhead radiant bed warmer. Children who have sustained thermal burns are at risk for hypothermia because the injured skin is no longer able to regulate body temperature.

17. The child is at risk for carbon monoxide poisoning, again because he was in a closed-space fire.

18. Carbon monoxide poisoning is diagnosed by a carboxyhemoglobin (COHb) level. Hemoglobin has a higher affinity for carbon monoxide than oxygen, so hemoglobin binds with carbon monoxide and prevents oxygen from binding and being transported. The child will not appear dusky or cyanotic, however, because carboxyhemoglobin is bright red.

19. Pulse oximetry cannot distinguish between oxyhemoglobin and carboxyhemoglobin, so pulse oximeters are not useful. A pulse oximeter reading is a combination of the hemoglobin bound to oxygen and the hemoglobin bound to carbon monoxide.

SUMMARY POINTS

1. Inhalation injury in children is the leading cause of morbidity and mortality in burn cases. Because the upper airways are extremely vascular, they attempt to remove heat from inhaled gases, thus producing edema. Pediatric airways are much smaller in diameter than adult airways, so edema has a much greater effect. Always assume an inhalation injury when the face or neck is burned, secretions from the nose or mouth are charred, or the child is unconscious.

2. It is extremely important to intubate early in the care of a child with an inhalation injury. Edema peaks 6 to 8 hours after exposure. An ETT one size smaller than usual may be needed if edema is already present.

3. Intraosseus lines are invaluable in emergencies when the child is in profound shock and access is necessary. They may, however, produce complications that require the line to be discontinued. Complications of intraosseous lines include infiltration, cellulitis, osteomyelitis, and epiphyseal plate damage. If one of these conditions occurs, remove the line and prepare to start one in another site.

4. After stabilizing airway and breathing, the child in shock requires immediate fluid resuscitation. Use non–glucose-containing fluids to avoid hyperglycemia and osmotic diuresis. Evaluate the effectiveness of fluid boluses after each bolus by checking the heart rate, capillary refill, peripheral pulses, and color and warmth of extremities.

5. The child with thermal burns > 40% of BSA requires two large bore IV or IO catheters and massive fluid resuscitation. Use the Parkland Formula to calculate the child's first 24 hour fluid requirements for burn injury. This amount is what the child needs from the time of the initial burn, not from the time the child is treated. Estimated fluid requirements according to the Parkland Formula are in addition to the child's maintenance fluid requirements. Consult burn specialists for guidance.

6. Carbon monoxide poisoning also may be present if the child was in a closed space fire; it is diagnosed by a carboxyhemoglobin level. A carboxyhemoglobin level >60% may be fatal. Carbon monoxide competes with oxygen for hemoglobin and thus produces hypoxia. Clinical signs and symptoms of hypoxia may not be present, however.

Case Study 3

◆ You receive in your ED a 2-year-old boy with two small puncture wounds to his left wrist. His mother reports that the child was playing in their back yard while she was hanging the laundry. He began crying, so she picked him up and took him inside. During his bath (15 minutes later), she noted the puncture wounds on his wrist. She became concerned and called the EMS system.

She did not see a snake, although she reports that her husband saw one a week ago in their backyard. She reports that the child's immunizations are up to date.

HR = 120 beats/minute   RR = 30 breaths/minute

BP = 110/65 mm Hg   T = 37.2° C rectally   Weight = 11.5 kg

1. What is your first priority?

◆ The child's respiratory rate is 30 breaths/minute and nonlabored. Breath sounds are clear to auscultation and slightly decreased in the bases. Skin is pink, warm, and dry. Upper extremity peripheral pulses are difficult to assess (he fusses when you touch him), but you think they are +1. Capillary refill is 3 seconds.

As you continue your assessment, you note the puncture wounds on the ventral side of his left wrist are reddened and ecchymotic. The ecchymosis extends approximately 2 cm around the wounds and his whole forearm is pink and swollen. Left wrist measures 14 cm. Right wrist measures 11 cm.

The physician requests lab work (serum electrolytes, CBC, and coagulation studies) and an IV.

2. Where is the best place to draw blood in this child?

3. Where do you start an IV in this child?

4. **What size over-the-needle catheter do you use to start an IV in this child?**

◆ You place an IV in his right hand with a 20 gauge catheter. You succeeded in obtaining blood samples for the lab work during the IV start.

5. **The physician requests $D_5^{1/4}NS$ at maintenance rate. What is maintenance rate for this child?**

◆ The child becomes increasingly fussy and splints his arm next to his body. There are no other changes in his vital signs or mental status. The left wrist measurement is now 15.5 cm. You are concerned that the child is in pain.

6. **What are signs and symptoms of pain in a child this age?**

7. **What can you do to help alleviate this child's pain?**

◆ The physician wrote transfer orders to the PICU for observation and possible antivenin infusion. She wrote an order for morphine 0.1 mg IV q2 to 4 hr prn.

8. **How do you check the dose of morphine?**

9. **What do you do?**

◆ The physician readily admits the dose is too low and rewrites the order as morphine 1 mg IV q2 to 4 hr prn.

You administer the medication and prepare to transport the child to the PICU.

SUGGESTED ANSWERS

1. As with any admission, start with the ABCs.

   a. Airway—Ensure that the airway is patent and stable.
   b. Breathing—After the airway is secured, assess for adequate ventilation. Assess respiratory rate and effort by observing the child's face, neck, and chest. Look for retractions, nasal flaring, and anxiety. Note his preferred position. Auscultate for breath sounds long the mid-axillary line. Severe envenomation could cause an anaphylactic-type reaction with airway difficulties. Other types of envenomation could lead

to pulmonary edema from injury of the pulmonary epithelial lining.

c. Circulation—After the airway is established and adequate ventilation is obtained, assess the circulatory status. Assess extremities for skin color, peripheral pulses, capillary refill, and temperature. Note the heart rate and blood pressure (if available). Certain types of venom cause changes in capillary membranes, which contribute to fluid extravasation and shock.

2. The antecubital fossa veins are ideal for drawing blood samples (see "Blood Sample Collection"). However, each child is different and veins in the hand or foot may also be used. If the child is chubby, the antecubital veins may be difficult to palpate. Avoid the affected extremity.

Since this child appears healthy, it may be possible to obtain enough blood samples for the labwork when starting an IV.

3. Veins in the dorsum of the hand, the foot, or in the antecubital fossa may be used. Use distal sites first. Avoid the affected extremity.

4. A 22, 20, or 18 gauge catheter may be used for children 1 to 12 years old.

5. See "Calculating Maintenance Intravenous (IV) Fluid Requirements." An hourly rate for this child is calculated by:

---

40 ml/hr for the first 10 kg plus
2 ml/hr for every kg over 10 kg

Therefore 40 ml/hr + 3 ml/hr = 43 ml/hr

---

6. Pain behaviors vary from child to child. Ask yourself, "Would a 'well' child be acting like this?" Parents may be able to tell you if behavior is "normal" for their child or not; however, they may not always be able to tell you if the child is in pain.

Children in pain may exhibit a wide variety of behaviors. Examples of pain behaviors for a 2-year-old include:

- restlessness
- aggressive behavior
- clinging to their caregiver
- refusal to move a body part
- crying
- tremors
- verbal stalling
- avoidance of eye contact
- inability to be easily distracted

7. A combination of pharmacologic and nonpharmacologic interventions is best. Appropriate analgesics for moderate to severe pain include morphine sulfate (0.1 to 0.2 mg/kg IV) or fentanyl (1 to 2 μg/kg IV). Both have a relatively rapid onset of action.

Nonpharmacologic interventions include:

- Keeping the parents with the child
- Preparing the child for experiences by explaining to him how it will feel
- Allowing the child some control
- Allowing the child as much movement as possible

8. Use a pediatric pharmacology reference manual. From *The Harriet Lane handbook,* the recommended dose of morphine for this child is 0.1 to 0.2 mg/kg/dose q2 to 4 hr prn.

The recommended dose range for this child (weight = 11.5 kg) is:

0.1 mg $\times$ 11.5 kg = 1.15 mg

0.2 mg $\times$ 11.5 kg = 2.3 mg

The dose of 0.1 mg IV q2 to 4 hr is extremely low compared to the recommended dose range.

9. Bring the dose to the physician's attention to determine if an error was made.

SUMMARY POINTS

1. Even though a snake bite can be frightening for both the child and the health care provider, always begin your assessment with the ABCs. Airway, breathing, and circulation *must* be stabilized before attending to the snake bite.

2. Intervention in the ED for a snake bite victim depends on several factors, including the symptoms present, the type of snake, and the time since the bite. Administration of antivenin depends on the grade of envenomation. Administration of antivenin may be given from 4 to 24 hours after the bite, although the greater the time between envenomation and antivenin therapy, the less effective the antivenin.

Determination of Severity of Envenomation and Therapy

Severity	Findings	Initial Therapy
None	Fang marks only; no local or systemic signs or symptoms	No skin test/antivenin
Minimal	Fang marks with slowly progressive local swelling; no systemic symptoms	5 vials (50 ml)
Moderate	History of multiple or provoked bites or bite of large venomous snake or highly toxic species (Mojave, diamondback); fang marks with edema rapidly progressing beyond the bite site; systemic symptoms including metallic taste, paresthesias; laboratory abnormalities	10 vials (100 ml)
Severe	History of bite of highly toxic snake, prolonged embedding of fangs, and multiple bites; fang marks with very rapidly progressive edema, subcutaneous hemorrhage; severe systemic reaction with muscle fasciculation, hypotension, oliguria; laboratory abnormalities	15 vials (150 ml)

Modified from Barkin RM et al, eds.: *Pediatric emergency medicine: concepts and clinical practice,* St Louis, 1992, Mosby, p. 405.

3. Although checking pediatric medication doses is time-consuming, it is imperative. The margin of error is small and the consequences may be great. Use a pediatric pharmacology reference manual. If a medication error is suspected, always bring it to the attention of the physician.

Case Study 4

◆ You receive in your ED a 3-month-old female respiratory arrested at home. The infant was sleeping and breathing when checked on at 3:00 AM today; when parents went back to check on her at 6:30 AM she was apneic. They began rescue breathing. The EMS system was alerted and responded.

When you receive the infant, CPR is being performed and a 3.0 mm ETT is in place orally. There is no venous access. Estimated weight by pediatric emergency tape is 4 kg.

The rescue squad transfers the infant to your stretcher and begins to give their report.

1. What is your first priority?

◆ In assessing the airway, you do not hear breath sounds in the mid-axillary area or any part of the chest.

2. What do you do?

◆ The infant is re-intubated orally with another 3.0 mm ETT. CPR continues.

3. What is the ideal depth for a 3.0 mm ETT in a 3 kg infant?

4. How do you tape the ETT?

5. What are your next priorities?

◆ CPR is appropriate with compressions at 100/minute and ventilation every fifth compression. A femoral pulse is palpated with each compression. When compressions are stopped, there are no spontaneous respirations and the heart rate is 30 beats/minute.

6. What is your next intervention?

217

7. How do you administer medication via the ETT? Which medications are appropriate for administering via the ETT?

◆ The epinephrine is unsuccessful in increasing the infant's heart rate.

8. What are your next interventions?

9. Where do you place an IO line?

10. What size IO needle do you use?

11. How do you insert the IO line?

12. How do you secure the IO line?

◆ A 15 gauge intraosseous (IO) needle is placed in the right tibia. A dose of epinephrine (0.04 mg) is given via the IO line. The heart rate fluctuates between 80 and 90 BPM, so CPR is stopped. The physician requests an epinephrine drip and a dose of sodium bicarbonate (ABG pending).

13. How do you mix an epinephrine drip for this infant?

◆ Despite your team's best efforts, the heart rate drops again to 40 beats/minute and progressively slows. Additional epinephrine doses do not produce a heartbeat. Resuscitation efforts are stopped and the infant is pronounced dead.

You and the physician prepare to inform the parents that their baby has died.

14. What specific interventions will assist the parents?

SUGGESTED ANSWERS

1. As with any admission, start with the ABCs.

    a. Airway—Ensure that the airway is patent and stable. Check ETT placement by auscultating over the mid-axillary line. If an end-title CO_2 device is available, confirm placement with it as well. Check the security of the tape on the ETT. Confirm patency of the ETT with the person who is ventilating.

    b. Breathing—After the airway is secured, assess for adequate ventilation. Observe chest excursion. Auscultate for breath sounds along the mid-axillary line. Observe skin color.

c. Circulation—After the airway is established and adequate ventilation is obtained, assess the circulatory status. During CPR, check the effectiveness of the compressions by palpating a femoral pulse.

2. Since the ETT is not correctly placed, it must be removed and replaced. Bag-valve-mask ventilate the infant while the team prepares for re-intubation (see "Bag-Valve-Mask Ventilation").

3. To estimate the depth to tape the ETT, use the following formula:

> ETT size $\times$ 3 = cm depth of insertion
>
> In this infant, the estimated depth is 9 cm (3 $\times$ 3).

4. See "Securing Pediatric Endotracheal Tubes (ETT)."

5. After the airway is secured, continue with assessment of the ABCs.

6. Continue CPR. Administer epinephrine via the endotracheal tube. The recommended dose per ETT is 0.1 mg/kg. The dose for this infant is 0.4 mg/kg. Use 1:1000 concentration of epinephrine when administering high doses.

7. See "Administering Medication Delivery via an Endotracheal Tube." Other medications appropriate for ETT administration are atropine, lidocaine, and naloxone.

8. a. Attempt an IO line to administer epinephrine.
   b. Continue CPR.

9. a. Tibial tuberosity site: 1 to 3 cm below the tibial tuberosity.
   b. Distal femur site: 2 to 3 cm above the external condyles.
   c. Medial malleolus site: Proximal to the medial malleolus and posterior to the saphenous vein.

10. Either a 15 or 18 gauge intraosseous needle, bone marrow needle, or spinal needle may be used for a 3-month-old infant.

11. See "Intraosseous (IO) Needle Insertion."

12. See "Securing an Intraosseous (IO) Needle."

13. For epinephrine, multiply the child's weight (kg) by 0.6. The product is the number of milligrams of medication to add to the buretrol to total 100 ml.

Then 1 ml/hr = 0.1 µg/kg/minute

Therefore 0.6 × 4 kg = 2.4 mg

This is the amount of epinephrine to add to the fluid in the buretrol to equal 100 ml. Then 1 ml/hr = 0.1 µg/kg/minute. See "Calculating Inotropic Infusions." Administer the inotrope on an infusion pump.

---

14. a. Tell them that their baby has died. Do not use phrases that may be less clear, such as "gone to heaven" or "passed away" or "is with the angels now."
   b. Assure the parents that everything possible was done to try to save their baby.
   c. Allow the parents as much time as they wish to spend with their baby. Provide for privacy.
   d. Assure the parents that there was nothing that they could have done to prevent the death of their baby. They may be feeling guilty about something they did or did not do.
   e. Enlist the aid of a grief specialist, social worker, or clergy to assist you and the family.

SUMMARY POINTS

1. Sudden infant death syndrome (SIDS) is the leading cause of death in children 1 month to 1 year of age. The peak incidence is between 2 and 4 months of age. Although is has been thoroughly researched, the exact etiology of SIDS remains unknown. SIDS cannot be determined in the ED; an autopsy is needed to confirm the diagnosis.

2. One of the most common causes of an ETT being dislodged is transferring the infant from one bed to another. *Always* check ETT placement after each transfer. Tape the ETT securely and recheck periodically.

3. The new American Heart Association recommendation
    for the endotracheal dose of epinephrine is 0.1 mg/kg.
    When administering high dose epinephrine, use the
    1:1000 concentration instead of 1:10,000 to avoid giving
    a large volume. Since studies of absorption after endo-
    tracheal administration of medications are extremely
    variable, IV/IO administration of epinephrine is always
    preferred over endotracheal delivery. Therefore always
    attempt venous access for delivery of epinephrine dur-
    ing an arrest.

4. Use the "rule of sixes" when mixing an inotropic infu-
    sion for an infant. Purge the line *after* the medication is
    added to the buretrol and thoroughly mixed so the
    inotrope is not delayed in reaching the patient.
    Administer the inotrope on an infusion pump.

5. Individual reactions to the death of a child vary and may
    include anger, hysteria, shock, guilt, or extreme calm. It
    is sometimes reassuring to the parents to know that
    "everything was done" for their child. Despite their ini-
    tial shock they often remember in detail the care they
    received in the ED. Enlist the aid of a grief specialist,
    social worker, or chaplain to assist you and the family
    during this critical time. Give the parents phone num-
    bers of local support groups, as well as the phone num-
    ber of someone in the ED that they can contact if they
    have questions later.

Case Study 5

◆ You receive in your ED a 4-year-old male who was the victim of a two-car motor vehicle crash. He was transported by the flight team. The child was found face down on the hood of a car involved in the head-on collision. It is not known how he arrived in that position. The driver of the vehicle was killed. The driver of the other vehicle was taken to a nearby hospital.

The child is fully immobilized on a pediatric immobilizer with head blocks and a cervical collar in place. The child is conscious and crying. He did not lose consciousness during the flight; it is unknown whether he lost consciousness at the scene of the accident.

The child is unable to open his eyes due to gross edema. Dried blood is noted in both nares but no drainage is noted from his ears or nose. His lips are swollen. The flight team reports that his two front teeth are broken off.

One 20 gauge IV is in place in his left antecubital fossa. O_2 is being administered by simple face mask. The child is resisting immobilization and the O_2 face mask.

HR = 150 beats/minute   RR = 20 breaths/minute
BP = 120/72 mm Hg

Estimated weight by pediatric emergency tape is 20 kg.

1. What is your first priority with this child?

◆ The child is able to maintain his airway without assistance. The child has clear and equal breath sounds bilaterally. Upper airway noises are audible. He is crying intermittently. His skin is warm, dry, and pale pink. Capillary refill is 3 seconds. Peripheral pulses are +2 in all four extremities.

No sites of active bleeding are noted on initial exam. An ecchymotic area (3 cm diameter) is noted on his forehead with gross periorbital and facial edema present.

2. How do you suction this child?

3. How do you administer oxygen (O_2) to this child?

◆ As you finish your primary survey, you note that the child has succeeded in wiggling his arms out of the immobilizer.

4. How do you immobilize this child?

5. How do you explain to the child what you are doing?

◆ As you are immobilizing him, you notice that his hands and feet are cool. You check the chart and see that his temperature has not been taken.

6. What is the most accurate method of taking a temperature for this child?

7. How do you explain this to the child?

◆ The child's temperature is 36.8° C per rectum. His hands and feet continue to be cool to the touch and capillary refill is now 4 to 5 seconds. He becomes more irritable with periods of lethargy.

HR = 145 beats/minute   BP = 110/72 mm Hg   RR = 12 breaths/minute

◆ The physician elects to intubate to protect the airway. As you are preparing for intubation, the child becomes apneic.

8. What do you do?

◆ While you are manually ventilating the child, you notice that it is becoming more difficult to obtain chest rise. Your colleague reports that his abdomen is becoming distended and offers to place an orogastric tube, since the child has potential facial fractures.

9. What size OG tube do you use?

10. How do you measure for placement?

11. How do you secure the OG tube?

◆ The OG is placed and the child's abdomen becomes softer and less distended. The child remains unconscious. Intubation with a 5.0 mm ETT is uneventful.

12. How do you tape an oral ETT?

13. How many breaths per minute do you manually ventilate for this child?

◆ Since the child is tachycardic and his color is pale, the physician requests a fluid bolus before the child is transported to the PICU.

14. How do you administer a fluid bolus to this child?

◆ The child remains stable as you prepare to transport him to CT scan and then to the PICU.

SUGGESTED ANSWERS

1. As with any admission, start with the ABCs.

    a. Airway—Ensure that the airway is patent and stable and institute cervical spinal immobilization. If the child cannot maintain an adequate airway, open the airway using the jaw thrust maneuver, assuming the child may have a cervical spine injury. Stand behind the child and place your hands on either side of his head; position your fourth and fifth fingers on the occiput and your second and third fingers along the mandible, forcing the mandible in an upward position (see "Bag-Valve-Mask Ventilation" and "Spinal Immobilization"). If necessary, suction any obvious secretions.

    b. Breathing—After the airway is secured, assess for adequate ventilation. Assess respiratory rate and effort by observing the child's face, neck, and chest. Look for retractions, nasal flaring, and anxiety. Note his preferred position. Observe chest excursion. Auscultate for breath sounds along the mid-axillary line. Observe skin color.

    c. Circulation—After the airway is established and adequate ventilation is obtained, assess the circulatory status. Assess extremities for skin color, peripheral pulses, capillary refill, and temperature. Note the heart rate and blood pressure (if available). Also check for any sites of active bleeding or ecchymosis.

2. Since he has dried blood in his nose and mouth and upper congestion but is conscious and crying, instruct the child to "spit out" the secretions in his mouth. If he is unable to do so, suction his mouth gently. Use a large bore (tonsil tip) catheter to suction the oropharyngeal area. Nasal suctioning is contraindicated because the child may have sustained a basilar skull fracture.

3. A simple face mask will deliver an O_2 concentration of 60% at 10 L/min and may be used if the child tolerates it. If he does not tolerate a face mask, use blow-by with 100% O_2 at 6 L/min. Nasal cannulae only provide an O_2 concentration of approximately 44% at 6 L/min. A flow rate higher than 6 L/min is irritating to the nasal mucosa. See "Administration of Oxygen (O_2)."

4. See "Spinal Immobilization." If the child is actively moving, two health care providers are needed, one to immobilize the head and neck and one to secure the child's body and head to the board.

   Use a cervical collar only if it is the right size, i.e. the chin fits in the groove without hyperextension or flexion and the sides of the collar do not cover his ears.

5. a. Explain immobilization by how it feels, not why you must do it. Give permission for him to wiggle his toes or fingers.

   EXAMPLE
   "Johnny, this is something that is going to help you hold really still. It might feel kind of tight for a while, but you can wiggle your toes and your fingers all you want. Let me see if you can wiggle your toes."

   b. Explain everything in simple, concrete terms. The preschooler thinks very literally; many medical terms may have a completely different meaning for him, such as "stretcher," "CAT scan," or "dye."
   c. Reassure him that he is *not* being punished and that the accident was not his fault. Preschoolers are obsessed with fairness.
   d. Offer abundant reassurances.

6. Take an initial rectal temperature with an electronic thermometer and correlate it with an axillary temperature. Axillary temperatures may then be used unless the temperature is abnormally high or low.

7. a. Explain the procedure right before you do it. Preschoolers do not have coping skills to deal with unpleasant events if told 5 to 10 minutes before the events happen.
   b. Explain to him how it will feel, not why you must do it. Explain in simple, concrete terms. Avoid saying, "Take your temperature" because you are not actually taking something from the child.
   c. Assure the child that he is not being punished.
   d. Offer abundant reassurances.

8. Begin bag-valve-mask ventilation for the child with the modified jaw-thrust maneuver to maintain airway control; this may require two people. Use a child-size mask and 500 ml resuscitation bag. See "Bag-Valve-Mask Ventilation."

9. Use a 10 F salem sump tube for a child weighing from 10 to 20 kg.

10. Measure from the nose to the earlobe to a point midway between the xyphoid process and the umbilicus.

11. See "Securing Nasogastric (NG) and Orogastric (OG) Tubes."

12. See "Securing an Endotracheal Tube (ETT)."

13. This child would normally require 20 breaths per minute; however, his injuries and sleepiness indicate a possible brain injury. Therefore hyperventilation is indicated.

    The endocranial vault contains three components: brain, blood, and cerebral spinal fluid. These elements are enclosed in a fixed system; when one component of the vault swells it is at the expense of another. Therefore if edema is occurring in the brain, vasoconstriction allows more room for the injured tissue. Hyperventilation produces vasoconstriction.

    Maintain the $PaCO_2$ between 25 and 30 mm Hg. Levels lower than this may produce cerebral ischemia. Begin manual ventilations at a rate of 30 to 35 breaths/minute, allowing adequate expiratory time. Obtain an ABG to determine the pH and $PaCO_2$.

14. Administer 20 ml/kg of LR according to "Intravenous (IV) Fluid Bolus Administration." Evaluate the heart rate, capillary refill, peripheral pulses, and color and temperature of extremities after the bolus.

SUMMARY POINTS

1. Establishing a patent airway and ensuring adequate oxygenation and ventilation are always the highest priority in any pediatric emergency. The jaw thrust maneuver is recommended in any child with suspected cervical spine injury.

2. Oxygen (100%) is always recommended in the acute phase of a pediatric trauma. While a nasal cannula may sometimes be tolerated better than a face mask, the cannula can only produce an oxygen concentration of approximately 44% at a flow rate of 6 L/min. Higher flow rates are irritating to the nasal mucosa. A face mask or blow-by provides a higher O_2 concentration.

3. In a child with head trauma and suspected increased intracranial pressure, it is important to establish a secured airway. Hyperventilate to prevent vasodilation of cerebral blood vessels, decrease the volume in the endocranial vault, and reduce intracranial pressure.

4. Immobilization with an active child requires two health care providers. One person is responsible for maintaining in-line cervical stabilization and communicating with the child. (Traction on the cervical area is no longer recommended.) The other person is responsible for immobilizing the body and head to the board. Immobilize the body first. In-line cervical stabilization can be discontinued only after both the body and the head are secured.

5. Preschoolers still have difficulty in distinguishing between fantasy and reality. They need clear and concrete explanations of what is happening. Since they do not fully understand cause and effect, focus on what the child will feel instead of the reason you must do a procedure.

   Preschoolers also are obsessed with fairness and will usually think that they have been bad or are being punished for something. Assure them that they are *not* being punished.

6. If the abdomen becomes distended with air during man-

ual ventilation, it impedes chest rise. This problem can be relieved by applying cricoid pressure to occlude the esophagus. Usually a gastric tube will need to be placed to relieve abdominal distention. While there are many techniques for measuring depth of insertion for a gastric tube, the recommended technique at present is to measure from the nose to the earlobe and then to a point between the xyphoid process and the umbilicus.

Case Study 6

◆ A mother brings her 4-year-old boy to your ED. She reports that he developed a fever this morning and is complaining of a sore throat. She is concerned because "he looks like he's having trouble breathing and acts scared."

You observe a very anxious child sitting up and leaning forward on his hands. His breathing is labored with suprasternal retractions, nasal flaring, and intercostal retractions.

1. How do you assess this child?

◆ Vital signs: HR = 130 beats/minute   RR = 28 breaths/minute

You summon a colleague to prepare intubation equipment and contact an anesthesiologist. The anesthesiologist suggests administering O_2 until she arrives.

2. How do you administer oxygen to this child?

◆ Suddenly the child becomes apneic and unresponsive. The monitor displays a heart rate of 60 beats/minute.

3. What do you do?

◆ You are able to ventilate this child with a resuscitator device. The heart rate fluctuates between 90 and 110 beats/minute. Two respiratory therapists arrive and continue ventilating for the child. The anesthesiologist also arrives to intubate. The child's estimated weight is 18 kg per pediatric emergency tape.

4. What equipment do you need for intubation?

5. The anesthesiologist is unable to see the larynx due to edema. What technique can assist her?

229

◆ The child is intubated orally with a 4.5 mm ETT. Breath sounds are clear and equal bilaterally. The respiratory therapists continue to ventilate at 20 breaths/minute.

6. How do you tape the ETT?

◆ The child remains stable as you prepare to transfer him to PICU.

SUGGESTED ANSWERS

1. a. Approach the child slowly and offer simple explanations. This child is displaying classic symptoms of epiglottitis. The child is already anxious because he is having difficulty breathing; be very careful not to create further anxiety. *Leave the child in his position of comfort and contact an anesthesiologist before assessing further.*

   b. Focus your assessment only on the priorities: airway, breathing, and circulation. *Do not attempt to look in his mouth.*

   c. Auscultate breath sounds and heart rate.

   d. Connect the child to a cardiorespiratory and pulse oximetry monitor.

   e. Do not leave the child unattended.

2. Administer O_2 by enlisting his mother's help; ask her to hold 100% blow-by O_2 near the child's nose and mouth. See "Administration of Oxygen (O_2)." Again, do not agitate the child.

3. Begin bag-valve-mask ventilation with a 500 ml resuscitation bag and a child mask. Use the chin lift–head tilt maneuver to open the airway. It may require two people to effectively ventilate this child. See "Bag-Valve-Mask Ventilation."

4. • ETT—probably a size smaller than usual for this child: 4.5, 5.0, 5.5 mm
   • Laryngoscope and blade—#2 straight or curved stylet
   • Suction catheter—Large bore to suction the oropharynx and an 8 to 10 F to suction the ETT
   • Tape
   • Benzoin
   • Povidone-iodine

- Medications: atropine (0.01 to 0.02 mg/kg)
             neuromuscular blocking agent
             sedative agent (fentanyl 1 to 2 µg/kg or
             midazolam 0.1 mg/kg)
- NG tube

Also obtain an emergency tracheostomy tray in the event intubation is unsuccessful.

5. Pressing down on the chest may produce a bubble that exits through the larynx; this will guide the anesthesiologist in visualizing the larynx and passing the ETT.

6. See "Securing an Endotracheal Tube (ETT)."

SUMMARY POINTS

1. Epiglottitis usually presents in children 2 to 6 years of age. It is characterized by sudden onset, high fever, drooling, and anxious appearance. These children often sit upright and lean forward to maximize their oxygen exchange.

2. It is very important to allow the child to remain in his or her position of comfort and to not agitate him or her. Keep interventions to a minimum and discontinue anything that upsets the child. Contact an anesthesiologist immediately and prepare to intubate.

3. If the child becomes apneic, bag-valve-mask ventilation may be effective with an adequate mask seal. This procedure requires two health care providers.

4. A stylet and an ETT one size smaller than usual may be required for intubation. After the ETT is placed, taping it securely is extremely important. Use a pulse oximeter and an end-title CO_2 device after intubation to assist in determining ETT placement.

Case Study 7

◆ You receive by ambulance a 2-year-old boy who was backed over by his parents' car. The EMS squad immobilized the toddler on an adult backboard but did not have an appropriate cervical collar to use.

A 4.0 mm ETT is in place orally and the EMS team has been hyperventilating the child at 30 breaths/minute. A 15 gauge IO needle is in his right tibia.

HR = 140 beats/minute   RR = 30 breaths/minute (bagging)
T = 35.0° C rectally

1. What is your first priority?

◆ Breath sounds are clear and equal bilaterally, with good air movement per manual ventilation. Extremities are pale; hands and feet are cool to touch with +1 peripheral pulses. Capillary refill is > 5 seconds.

2. Your colleague places an infant cervical collar on the child. How do you know if it is an appropriate size for this toddler?

◆ The physician requests a fluid bolus of LR to improve the child's poor perfusion.

3. How do you administer a fluid bolus to this child?

◆ You are concerned because the child's temperature is low and his peripheral perfusion is poor.

4. How do you warm this child?

◆ As you are adjusting the radiant warmer, your colleague administers another fluid bolus per the physician's request. Extremities are now pale pink with 3 to 4 second capillary refill. Hands and feet are warming. Peripheral pulses remain +1. Respiratory therapy continues to manually ventilate via the ETT. An ABG has been sent.

5. **To monitor the effectiveness of the fluid boluses, you decide the child needs a urinary catheter. What size catheter do you use for this child?**

6. **The catheter is placed without difficulty. How do you secure the catheter?**

◆ The child remains stable as you prepare for transport to CT scan and admission to the intensive care unit.

SUGGESTED ANSWERS

1. As with any admission, start with the ABCs.

   a. Airway—In a trauma victim, assessment of the airway and cervical spine immobilization are performed simultaneously. Ensure that the airway is patent and stable. Check ETT placement by auscultating over the mid-axillary line. If an end-title CO_2 device is available, confirm placement with it as well. Remember that a common cause of ETT dislodgement is transferring the child from the stretcher to the bed. Confirm patency of the ETT with the person who is ventilating.

   b. Breathing—After the airway is secured, assess for adequate ventilation. Observe chest excursion. Auscultate for breath sounds along the mid-axillary line. Observe skin color.

   c. Circulation—After the airway is established and adequate ventilation is obtained, assess the circulatory status. Assess extremities for skin color, peripheral pulses, capillary refill, and temperature. Note the heart rate and blood pressure (if available). Also check for any sites of active bleeding or ecchymosis.

2. The child's chin should fit snugly in the groove of the collar. If his chin is hyperextended or flexed, do not use the collar. The collar should not cover the child's ears.

3. Administer 20 ml/kg of LR according to "Intravenous (IV) Fluid Bolus Administration." Evaluate the heart rate, capillary refill, peripheral pulses, and color and temperature of extremities after the bolus.

4. Since the child will need stabilization procedures and observation, use a radiant bed warmer. An overhead radiant bed warmer will fit over the child's bed and still allow access to the child (see "Using Radiant Warmers").

5. An 8 to 10 F catheter is appropriate for a 2-year-old (see "Placing an Indwelling Urinary Catheter").

6. See "Securing an Indwelling Urinary Catheter."

SUMMARY POINTS

1. Opening the airway and cervical spinal immobilization are performed simultaneously in the pediatric trauma victim. Secure both the child's head and body to a backboard; if an appropriate cervical collar is not available, use towel rolls to immobilize.

2. Infants and children have difficulty maintaining their body temperature. Cold stress increases metabolic rate and oxygen consumption; if unresolved it can lead to metabolic acidosis. Use an overhead radiant warmer if the child requires constant observation and resuscitation interventions.

3. Urine output measurement is indicative of end-organ perfusion and evaluates the effectiveness of volume resuscitation. A urinary catheter is used to evaluate perfusion and fluid resuscitation for the child in shock. Secure the catheter to prevent it from being dislodged or causing trauma to the urethra.

Case Study 8

◆ A 16-year-old female presents in your ED with complaints of abdominal pain. She thinks she might be pregnant but has not seen a physician about it. She doesn't remember when her last menstrual period was; she reports that her periods have never been regular. She has no other major health problems.

On examination, the infant's head is crowning and vaginal discharge is bloody. You do not see any meconium.

1. What do you do?

◆ Within minutes an infant boy is born. You begin suctioning the infant's mouth and nose with a bulb syringe. The infant begins to breathe spontaneously and his color becomes pink. You clamp the umbilical cord.

HR = 160 beats/minute   RR = crying

2. For what condition is this newborn now at risk?

3. How can you prevent this?

4. What is the most appropriate method for taking a temperature in this newborn?

◆ The newborn's temperature is 36.0° C rectally. You suspect the newborn is slightly premature and so request an isolette to warm him while you prepare transport to an institution with a nursery.

5. How do you preheat the isolette?

6. How do you regulate the "air temperature" based on the infant's temperature?

SUGGESTED ANSWERS

1. Prepare for delivery and newborn resuscitation. Transport to another facility is not feasible as delivery is imminent. Obtain a delivery kit and a bed warmer or isolette.

   Risk factors for this delivery include the young age of the mother, the lack of prenatal care, and the potential premature age of the newborn.

2. Newborns are at risk for hypothermia immediately after birth. They have moved from a warm internal environment to a very cool environment where heat loss from conduction, convection, and evaporation occurs quickly. They also have limited resources for maintaining their body temperatures. Hypothermia increases metabolic rate and oxygen consumption; if unresolved it will lead to metabolic acidosis and death.

3. Thoroughly dry the newborn and remove the wet towels. Swaddle the newborn with dry towels. Turn up the heat in the room, if possible, and obtain an isolette or radiant bed warmer.

4. Take a rectal temperature using an electronic thermometer. Doing so measures the core temperature and also rules out anal atresia for the newborn. After an initial rectal temperature, axillary temperatures are appropriate.

5. Before placing the newborn in the isolette, preheat the linens and the inside by setting the "control temperature" to 37.0° C. When the "air temperature" reaches 37.0° C, unwrap the infant and place him inside the isolette (see "Using an Isolette").

6. Attach the isolette's temperature probe to the newborn's abdomen with the metal side against his body. Cover the probe with a reflective cover. Set the "control temperature" to 36.5° C; doing so will now regulate the temperature inside the isolette to maintain the newborn's skin temperature at 36.5° C (see "Using an Isolette").

   Continue to monitor the newborn's axillary temperature after he is in the isolette.

SUMMARY POINTS

1. After assessment and stabilization of the ABCs with a newborn, provide measures to prevent hypothermia. Newborns lack the ability to shiver and cannot maintain their body temperatures. Cold stress increases metabolic rate and oxygen consumption. If unresolved, this leads to acidosis and shock.

2. Isolette warming is appropriate for the stable newborn. Regulate the isolette according to the operator's manual. Preheating the isolette decreases the newborn's heat loss; using the temperature probe regulates the isolette temperature according to the newborn's thermoregulation needs.

Case Study 9

1. Prepare a 3-year-old for IV insertion.

2. Prepare a 6-year-old for a CT scan with and without contrast.

3. Prepare a 4-year-old for suturing of her leg wound.

4. Prepare a 7-year-old for a urine specimen collection.

5. Describe the following medical terms or choose other phrasing for discussion with a 5-year-old.

   a. "to the floor"
   b. "PICU"
   c. "stool collection"
   d. "IV"
   e. "stretcher"
   f. "put you to sleep"
   g. "deaden"
   h. "take your vital signs"

SUGGESTED ANSWERS

> NOTE: THE EXAMPLES GIVEN FOR THESE SCENARIOS ARE MERELY SUGGESTIONS TO FACILITATE DISCUSSION. SEVERAL OPTIONS ARE ACCEPTABLE. SEE THE DEVELOPMENTAL GUIDELINES (CHAPTER 5) FOR ADDITIONAL INFORMATION.

1. "I need to put this small bendable tube in your arm. I will use a needle. It will pinch at first. Some children say it feels like a prick or a sting. But then I will take the needle out and throw it away. You can scream and cry if you want, but you can't kick or bite. I need you to try to hold this arm real still."

2. "We're going to take pictures of your [head] with a big

machine. You'll lie on a bed and the machine is like a big doughnut around your head. When I tell you, you'll need to lie real still. After the first picture, I'll put some medicine in this plastic tube in your arm. The medicine might sting. Then you'll need to let the machine take another picture."

3. "I'm going to fix the owie you have in your leg. You're going to feel a sting at first. After the stinging, your owie won't feel anything. The doctor will stitch the owie, but you shouldn't feel it then."

4. *(Find out from the parent what words the child uses for urine, voiding, and perineum.)*

   "I need to put some of your [pee] in this bottle so we can make sure you're okay. I will wipe your [bottom] and then you need to try to [pee] in this bottle."

5. a. "to another unit in the hospital"
   b. "to a part of the hospital where the nurses and doctors can take special care of you"
   c. Find out the child's familiar word.
   d. "a bendable tube in your arm so we can give you medicine through it"
   e. "bed with wheels"
   f. "give you medicine that will make you go to sleep; you won't feel anything while you're asleep and when you wake up the [operation] will be over"
   g. "give you medicine that will make your owie not feel anything"
   h. "measure your temperature and listen to your heart"

APPENDIX

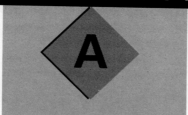

A

Abbreviations

ABC	airway-breathing-circulation
ABG	arterial blood gas
BP	blood pressure
BSA	body surface area
C°	Celsius
CBC	complete blood count
cc	cubic centimeter
COHb	carboxyhemoglobin
CPR	cardiopulmonary resuscitation
CT	computed tomography
DOB	date of birth
ED	emergency department
EL	esophageal length
EMS	emergency medical service
ETT	endotracheal tube
F°	Fahrenheit
F	French
Hg	mercury
hr	hour(s)
HR	heart rate
IO	intraosseus

IV	intravenous
kg	kilograms
L	liter
lbs	pounds
LR	lactated ringer's solution
mg	milligrams
min	minute
ml	milliliters
NG	nasogastric
NS	normal saline
O_2	oxygen
OG	orogastric
$PaCO_2$	arterial carbon dioxide tension
PaO_2	arterial oxygen tension
PEEP	positive end-expiratory pressure
PICU	pediatric intensive care unit
pO_2	partial pressure of oxygen
prn	as needed
Q	every
RR	respiratory rate
SIDS	sudden infant death syndrome
s/p	status post
T	temperature
U	units
VP	ventriculoperitoneal
μg	micrograms

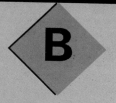

A P P E N D I X

B

Normal Vital Signs in Children

B

Normal Heart Rates in Children*

Age	Awake heart rate (per min)	Sleeping heart rate (per min)
Neonate	100-180	80-160
Infant (6 mo)	100-160	75-160
Toddler	80-110	60-90
Preschooler	70-110	60-90
School-age child	65-110	60-90
Adolescent	60-90	50-90

*Always consider patient's normal range and clinical condition. Heart rate will normally increase with fever or stress. Adapted from Gillette PC et al: Dysrhythmias. In Adams FH and Emmanouilides GC (eds): *Moss' heart disease in infants, children, and adolescents,* ed 4, Baltimore, 1989, Williams & Wilkins.

Normal Respiratory Rates in Children*

Age	Rate (breaths per min)
Infant	30-60
Toddler	24-40
Preschooler	22-34
School-age child	18-30
Adolescent	12-16

*Your patient's normal range should always be considered. Also, the child's respiratory rate is expected to increase in the presence of fever or stress.

Modified from Hazinski MF: *Nursing care of the critically ill child,* ed 2, St. Louis, 1992, Mosby.

Normal Blood Pressure in Children*

Age	Systolic pressure (mm Hg)	Diastolic pressure (mm Hg)
Birth (12 hr, <1000 g)	39-59	16-36
Birth (12 hr, 3 kg weight)	50-70	25-45
Neonate (96 hr)	60-90	20-60
Infant (6 mo)	87-105	53-66
Toddler (2 yr)	95-105	53-66
School-age child (7 yr)	97-112	57-71
Adolescent (15 yr)	112-128	66-80

*Blood pressure ranges taken from the following sources: *Neonate:* Versmold H et al: Aortic blood pressure during the first 12 hours of life in infants with birth weight 610-4220 gms, *Pediatrics* 67:107, 1981. 10th to 90th percentile ranges used. *Others:* Horan MI, chairman: Task Force on Blood Pressure Control in Children, report of the Second Task Force on Blood Pressure in Children, *Pediatrics* 79:1, 1987. 50th to 90th percentile ranges indicated.

Modified from Hazinski MF: *Nursing care of the critically ill child,* ed 2, St. Louis, 1992, Mosby.

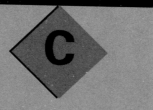

A P P E N D I X

C

Pediatric Coma Scale

NEUROLOGIC ASSESSMENT

Pupils	Right	Size	
		Reaction	
	Left	Size	
		Reaction	

++ = Brisk
+ = Sluggish
− = No reaction
C = Eye closed by swelling

Pupil scale (mm)
• 1
• 2
● 3
● 4
● 5
● 6
● 7
● 8

Eyes open	Spontaneously	4	
	To speech	3	
	To pain	2	
	None	1	

Usually record best arm or age-appropriate response

Best motor Response	Obeys commands	6	
	Localizes pain	5	
	Flexion withdrawal	4	
	Flexion abnormal	3	
	Extension	2	
	None	1	

Best response to auditory and/or visual stimulus	>2 years			<2 years
	Orientation	5		5 Smiles, listens, follows
	Confused	4		4 Cries, consolable
	Inappropriate words	3		3 Inappropriate persistent cry
	Incomprehensible words	2		2 Agitated, restless
	None	1		1 No response
	Endotracheal tube or trach	T		
Coma Scale Total				

Redrawn from Wong DL: *Pediatric quick reference,* St. Louis, 1991, Mosby, p. 14.

GLASGOW COMA SCALE

C

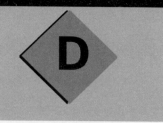
Instructor Guidelines

The instructor guidelines are written for nurses who teach other nurses either in a formal setting (e.g., unit educators, classroom instructors) or an informal setting (e.g., preceptorships). They outline the manual and offer suggestions to the instructor for using this pocket guide as a teaching tool.

The purpose of this manual is to provide well-illustrated and thorough guidelines for the performance of nursing procedures for infants and children. The manual is written for emergency department nurses, clinic nurses, transport nurses, pediatric nurses, students of nursing, and nurses who may infrequently care for pediatric patients.

NOTE: Before performing any procedure, a nurse should be familiar with her or his institution's policy and procedure manual, as well as the state's Nurse Practice Act. Although this manual offers guidelines based on relevant research, the policies and procedures of the individual institutions must be followed. These guidelines may help revise older policies or may serve as standards where written policies are not available.

The manual consists of two main parts:

A. guidelines for specific pediatric procedures
B. case studies to stimulate discussion and allow demonstration of the techniques.

A. PEDIATRIC PROCEDURE GUIDELINES

The guidelines are divided into five main sections:
1. Venous Access
2. Fluids and Medications
3. Oxygenation and Ventilation
4. Stabilization Procedures
5. Developmental Issues

Each guideline is written in stepwise format to facilitate learning for the beginner. The guidelines are written in the following format: (1) purpose; (2) supplies; and (3) procedure. Illustrations clarify and emphasize difficult steps. The experienced learner will benefit from the documentation of specific steps in current research and from highlighting the differences in certain steps between adult and pediatric techniques.

For example, when teaching "Peripheral Intravenous (IV) Cannulation," it is important for the instructor to highlight the steps specific to pediatrics since more health care providers will know the basic steps of peripheral IV cannulation. Instead of reading through the beginning steps of the guideline, for example, the instructor should highlight and discuss the parts of Step 2 that are specific to pediatrics.

PROCEDURE

1. Assemble IV infusion setup and purge with the IV fluids ordered.

   - Ensure that there are no bubbles in the tubing.
   - Label the bag and tubing with date and time.
   - Place the end of tubing within easy reach.

2. Assemble cannulation supplies. Keep needles out of sight of the child.

   - Flush the T-connector with normal saline or heparin solution.
   - Ensure that there are no bubbles in the T-connector.
   - Place the T-connector within easy reach to immediately attach it to the catheter hub.

   The use of a T-connector decreases movement and tension on the catheter and allows for IV tubing to be changed without disturbing the dressing or manipulating the catheter.[1,2]

3. Cut tape in 1 cm × 5 cm pieces for securing the IV catheter.
4. Procure assistance to restrain the infant or child.

When teaching the guidelines, demonstrate all techniques, eemphasizing the pediatric-specific steps. After the instructor has demonstrated the techniques, it is important that the learners also demonstrate the skills. The skills may also be demontrated in combination with the case studies.

Developmental Considerations

Each guideline instructs the learner to prepare the child for he procedure according to the child's developmental level and to provide positive feedback to the child after the procedure. *All procedures are difficult for children.* Children may not behave perectly during a procedure, but they need to be reassured that they "performed well" during the procedure. Emphasize positive behavior, regardless of the child's age.

For example, Steps 5 to 7 in "Peripheral Intravenous (IV) Cannulation" instruct the learner in preparing the child and parents for the intervention. Again, any procedure, particularly if it involves needles, is difficult for children. Highlight and discuss Steps 5 and 7.

5. Explain to the child and family the need for IV cannulation.

  • Be careful in your choice of words; for example, "IV" may be interpreted as "ivy" by the child.
  • Explain that you will put "a small tube in your arm" and that a needle is used in the beginning and then taken out and thrown away.
  • Be honest (tell the child that it will hurt and you will try to do it quickly).
  • If the child is 2 to 7 years old, tell him or her right before you are ready to start.
  • If the child is older and time permits, tell him or her 5 to 10 minutes before the cannulation attempt.

6. Ask a parent if the child has any known allergies (e.g., antiseptics, tape, medications).

D

7. Offer parents the option of staying for the procedure or waiting outside.
   Some parents may need permission to leave. If they do stay, their role is to offer support, not to restrain the child.

8. Wash hands.

Complete developmental guidelines are in Chapter 5. The: guidelines elaborate on behaviors of each age group and off ideas for the health care provider working with children. They a designed to be incorporated into each procedure as appropriate

B. PEDIATRIC CASE STUDIES

Nine case studies are located in Chapter 6. The case studies a designed to integrate the didactic knowledge with skills perfo mance. Case study questions are intended to stimulate discussic and to encourage return demonstration of the skills by the lear er. The case studies exemplify application of the procedures.

The four parts of the case study format are explained below.

1. Patient scenario

Each case study begins with a patient scenario.

◆ You receive in your emergency department (ED) a 4-year-old male with a history of hydrocephalus s/p a VP shunt placement shortly after birth. Mother reports that the child woke up this AM with a high fever and she has been unable to bring it down with acetaminophen.

Objective assessment reveals a lethargic boy who responds to speech but is content to lie quietly on the exam bed. Estimated weight by the pediatric emergency tape is 13 kg.

HR = 150 beats/minute RR = 24 breaths/minute T = 39.5° C rectally (You cannot locate a blood pressure cuff in the right size and therefore are unable to obtain a blood pressure reading.)

D

2. Question format

The questions that follow the patient scenario are either knowledge questions or action questions. Knowledge questions ask the learner for specific didactic information.

1. What is your first priority?

Action questions request a demonstration.

3. How do you explain to the child what you will be doing?

9. How do you secure the IV in his left hand?

Patient information needed to complete the case study is provided before relevant questions.

◆ The child's airway is uncompromised and he is breathing without effort at 24 breaths/minute. No retractions or nasal flaring noted. Breath sounds are clear and equal bilaterally, decreased in bases.

Apical heart rate is strong and regular at 150 beats/minute; S_1 and S_2 present without murmur. Extremities are pink and hot with 2 second capillary refill. Peripheral pulses are +2 in all four extremities.

3. Answer format

Answers are printed at the end of each case study. The didactic information is for the instructor to expound on.

1. As with any admission, start with the ABCs.

    a.   Airway—Ensure that the airway is patent and stable. If necessary, open the airway and suction any obvious secretions.

    b.   Breathing—After the airway is secured, assess for adequate ventilation. Assess respiratory rate and effort by observing the child's face, neck, and chest. Look for retractions, nasal flaring, and anxiety. Note child's preferred position. Auscultate for breath sounds along the mid-axillary line. Observe skin color.

D

c. Circulation—After the airway is established and adequate ventilation is obtained, assess the circulatory status. Assess extremities for skin color, peripheral pulses, capillary refill, and temperature. Note the heart rate and blood pressure (if available).

When teaching, encourage the learner to ask for patient information rather than offering the information freely.

Questions that ask the learner how to perform a particular skill encourage return demonstration. The answers to these skills questions refer to the guideline for that skill; this is done to avoid redundancy, not merely to read the answer to the learner. Encourage the learner to demonstrate the skill, using the guideline if needed.

9. See "Securing IV Catheters."

4. Summary points

All case studies end with a summary emphasizing important points.

SUMMARY POINTS

1. Drawing blood samples and starting IVs in children is often a difficult task. Selecting the most accessible site offers the greatest chance of success. The antecubital fossa is the site of choice for drawing blood samples. For children 3 years and older, veins in the dorsum of the hand or the antecubital fossa may be used for IV insertion.

    If the child has a chronic condition that has required numerous blood draws or IV insertions, the parents may be able to identify previous successful sites.

2. Although checking pediatric medication doses is time-consuming, *it is imperative.* The margin of error is small and the consequences may be great. Use a pediatric pharmacology reference manual

and consult with the physician if the dose is inappropriate.

C. Integration of Guidelines and Case Studies

When teaching in a classroom setting, use skills stations to offer the opportunity for hands-on practice. The skills stations can be combined as station 1 (venous access, fluids and medications); station 2 (oxygenation and ventilation); and station 3 (stabilization procedures, developmental issues). See the table below.

Skills station	Guidelines
1	Venous access
	Fluids and medications
2	Oxygenation and ventilation
3	Stabilization procedures
	Developmental issues

Set up stations for small group discussion of case studies after all learners have attended the skills stations.

Allow $1^1/_2$ to 2 hours for each skills station, depending on the pediatric experience of the learners. Demonstration and teaching of the guidelines generally require 45 to 60 minutes. Case study stations for return demonstration and discussion may require 60 to 90 minutes for 3 to 4 case studies.

D. Equipment needed

Procuring enough equipment may be difficult and time-consuming; however, it greatly enhances the learner's experience. Equipment needed for each skills station is listed below.

1. Skills station 1: Venous access, fluids and medications

Pediatric IV arm or scalp training mannequin
Pediatric IO leg training mannequin
Nonsterile gloves
Alcohol pads
Povidone-iodine solutions
Nonsterile 2" × 2" gauze pads
Sterile adhesive bandage strips
23 or 25 gauge butterfly needle
Four 10 ml syringes
Blood collection tubes

Heparinized syringe
Tourniquet or rubber band
Microlancet
Capillary tubes
Clay sealer
24, 22, or 20 gauge over-the-needle catheter
T-connector
1/4" to 1/2" adhesive tape
Padded armboard
Transparent dressing
Cotton
Sterile 2" × 2" gauze
Intraosseous needles
2" to 3" IV extension tubing
Three-way stopcock
60 ml syringe
Sterile 4" × 4" gauze pads
3" conforming gauze bandage
Kelly clamp
IV fluid
IV infusion setup
IV extension tubing
IV connecting tubing
Pediatric emergency tape
Pediatric pharmacology reference manual
Emergency medications

2. Skills station 2: Oxygenation and ventilation

Pediatric intubation head training mannequin
Infant mannequin
Bag-valve-mask ventilation device (500 ml)
Nasal cannula
Simple oxygen mask
Partial or non-rebreathing mask
Infant mask
Child mask
Nasogastric tube (8 to 10 F)
Endotracheal tubes (3.0 mm to 5.0 mm)
Suction catheters (6 to 12 F)
Secretion trap
Water-soluble lubricant
1/2" adhesive tape
Benzoin
Alcohol pads
Nonsterile gauze

Endotracheal medications (epinephrine 1:1000, atropine,
  lidocaine, naloxone)
Two 3 ml syringes
5 F feeding tube
Sterile gloves
Pediatric emergency tape

3. Skills station 3: Stabilization procedures

Child mannequin
Long backboard
Towel rolls
Semi-rigid cervical collar (infant and child size)
1$\frac{1}{2}$" to 2" adhesive tape
Thermometer (mercury or electric)
Nonsterile gloves
Water-soluble lubricant
Nasogastric tubes (8 to 12 F)
$\frac{1}{2}$" adhesive tape
20 ml syringe
Sterile gloves
Urinary catheters (5 to 10 F)
10 ml syringe
Cotton balls
Povidone-iodine solution
Urinary drainage set
Pediatric emergency tape

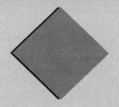

Index

A

B

C